Why Replace a Missing Back Tooth?

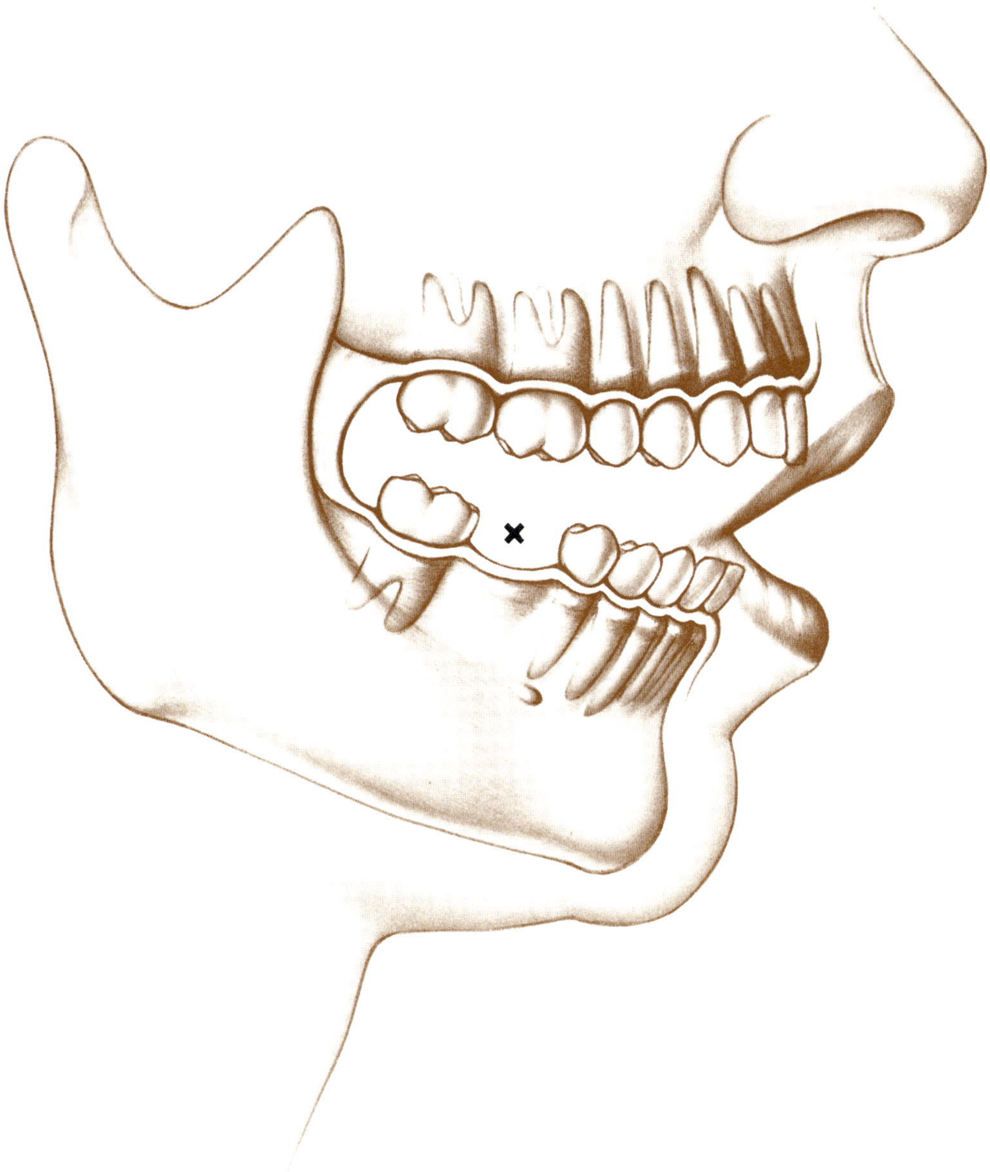

Library of Congress Cataloging in Publication Data

Berns, Joel M.
Why replace a missing back tooth?

1. Prosthodontics—Popular works. I. Title.
RK651.B38 1984 617.6′9 84-13455
ISBN 0-86715-135-8

quintessence books

Art and text by Explanatory Publications (Joel M. Berns, D.M.D.)
Illustrations: John Karapelov

Lithography and composition: The Clarinda Co., Clarinda, IA
Printing and binding: Christian Board of Publication, St. Louis, MO
Printed in U.S.A.

If you fail to replace an extracted back tooth with a false tooth, you could lose all of your teeth. This booklet explains how.

This booklet contains general principles. There are individual exceptions.

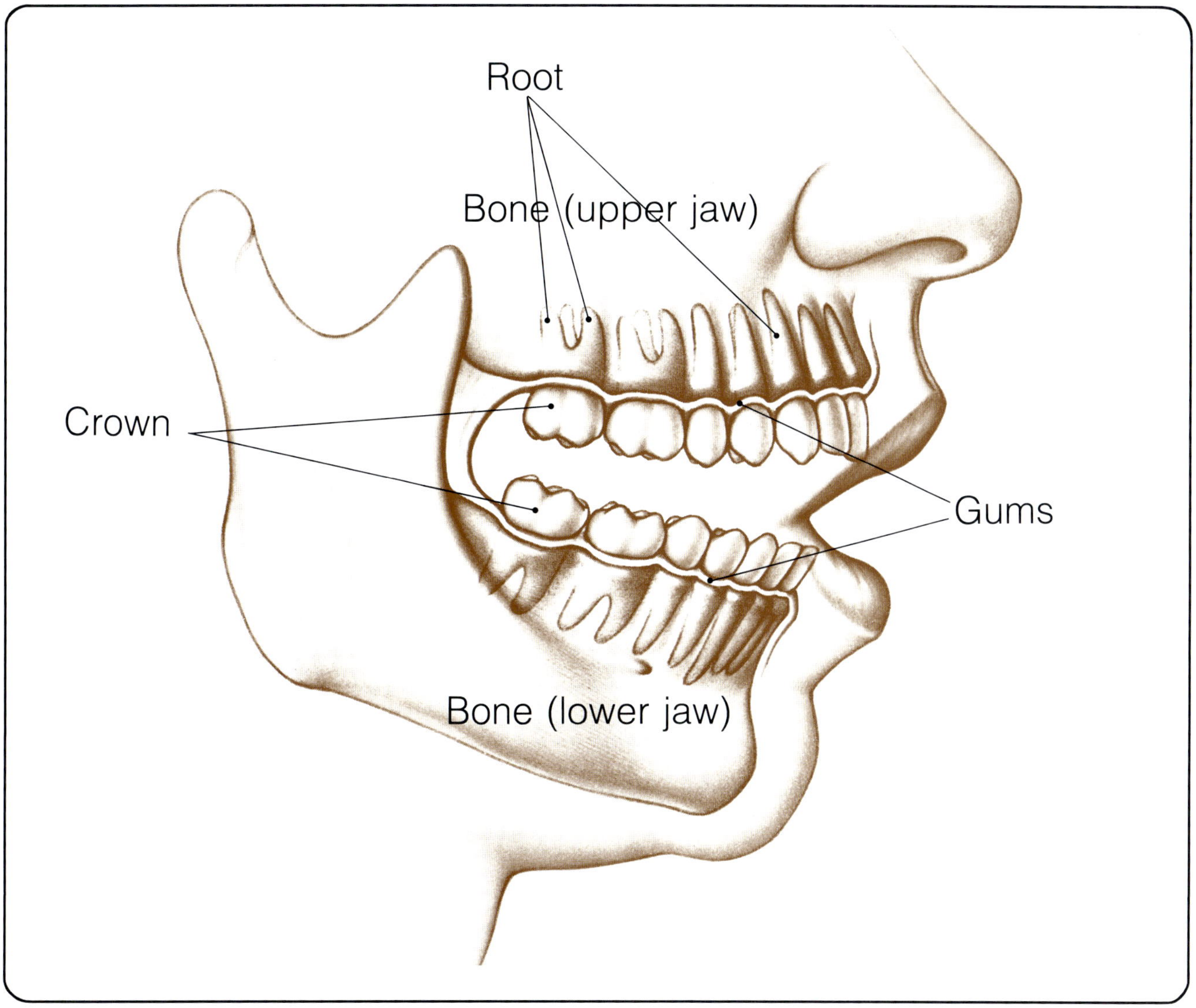

ANATOMY

Each tooth consists of two parts: the *crown* and the *root(s)*.

Only the crown is visible in the mouth. The roots are in the bone, under the gums.

The *gums* are a protective type of skin that clings to the necks of the teeth and covers the bone holding the teeth.

Molars are back teeth. They have two or three roots. Most other teeth have one root.

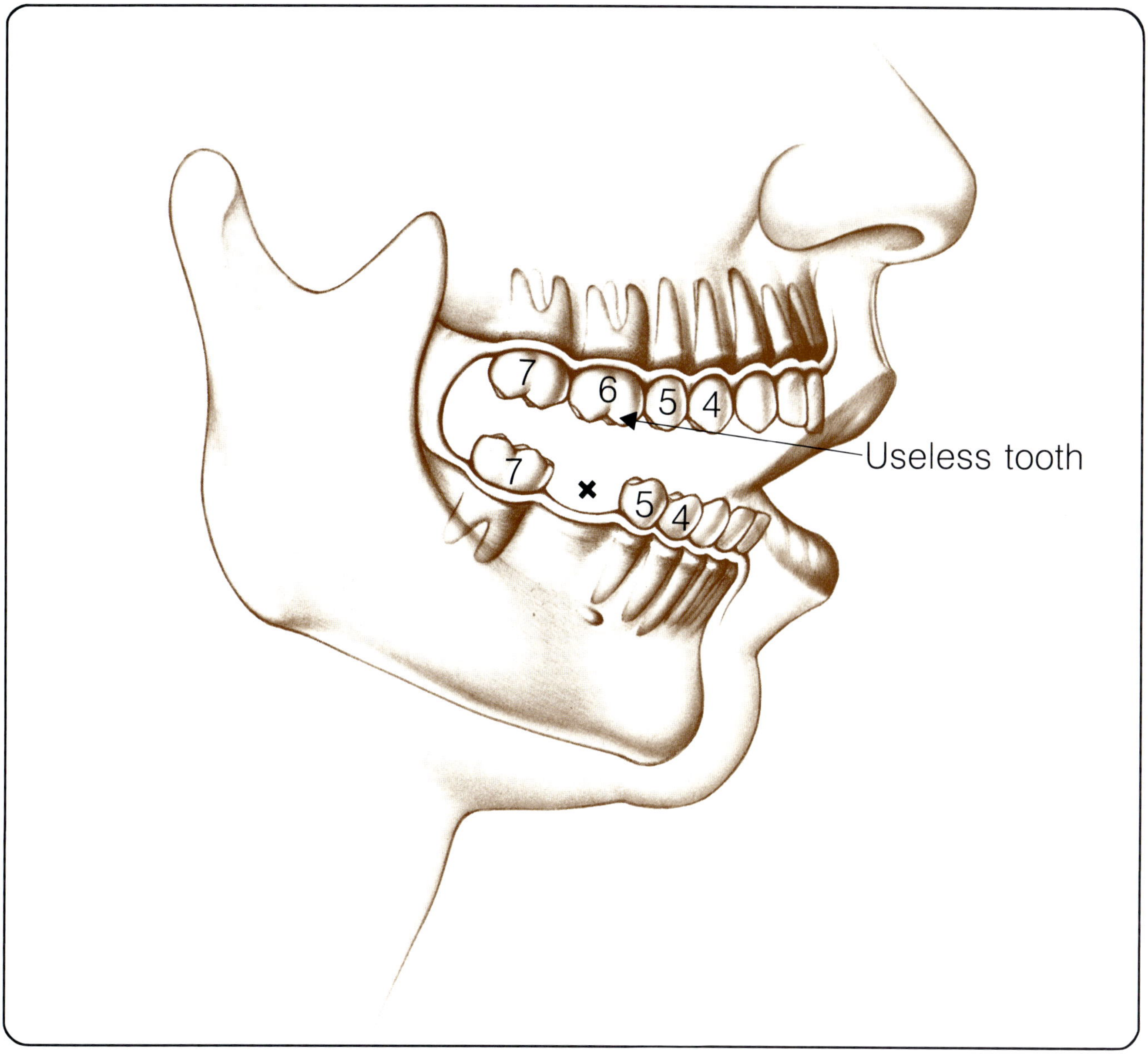

LOSING TEETH "TWO-FOR-ONE"

Recent extraction of a lower molar has created space X. Upper tooth 6 is now useless because it no longer has a tooth to chew against.

Therefore, *losing one tooth can result in the loss of the use of two*. Losing two teeth can result in the loss of the use of four, and so on.

A series of problems begins

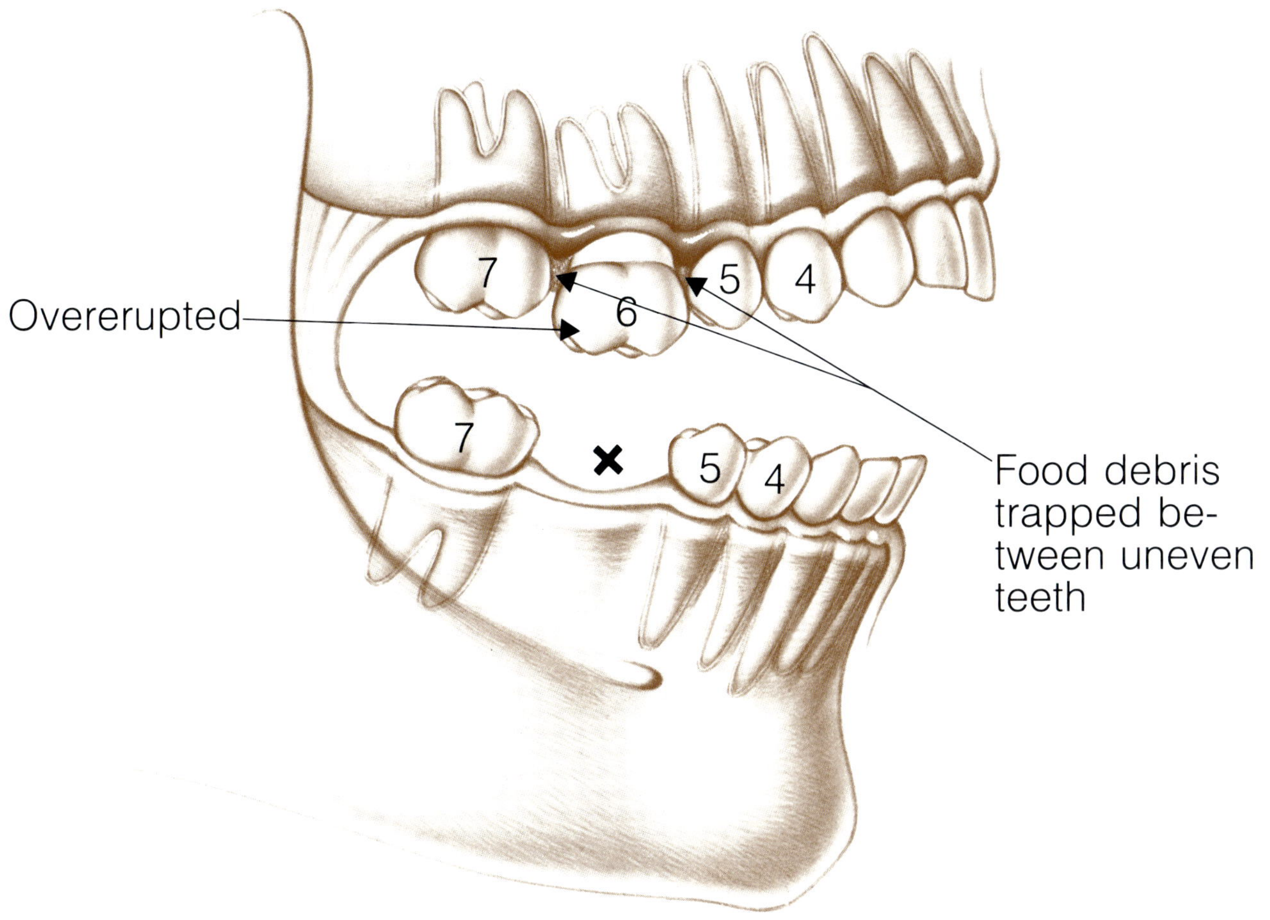

OVERERUPTION

Back teeth have a lifetime tendency to *erupt* (move farther into the mouth). Only the presence of a tooth to chew against keeps a back tooth from *overerupting*.

This patient had a tooth extracted from space X. Upper tooth 6 has overerupted.

The resulting unevenness among the upper back teeth has created areas between these teeth that trap debris. It is very difficult to keep spaces between uneven teeth clean, despite your best efforts at brushing and flossing.

Unclean teeth usually cause inflammation of the surrounding gums. They decay more readily too.

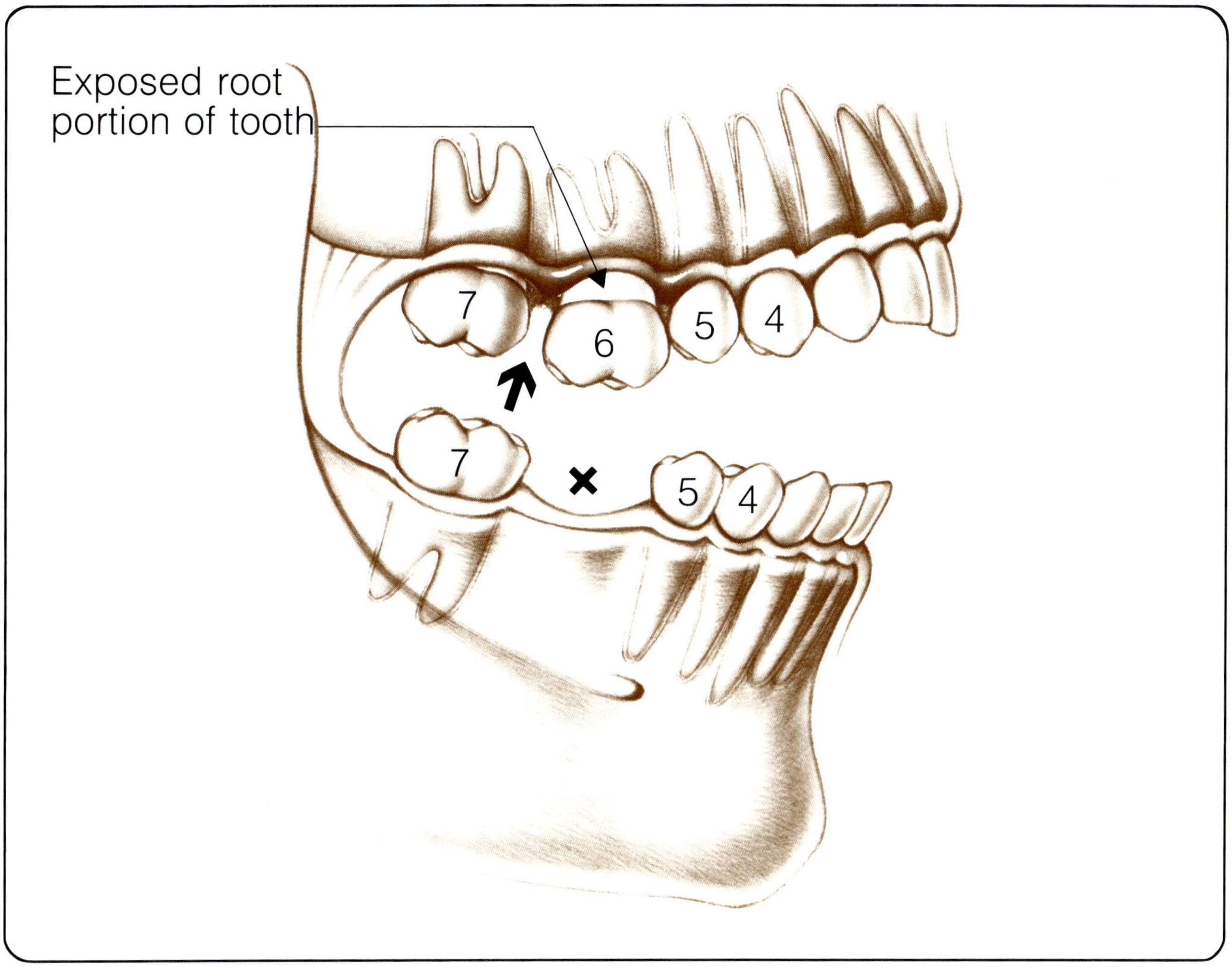

Lower molar 7 is jamming food in between overerupted 6 and 7 during eating (arrow).

This pressure between upper 6 and 7 has caused upper 7 to move backward and separate slightly from upper 6. It has created a space between these teeth (arrow). Food can pack into this space with great force during chewing. This creates a serious inflammation of the gum.

Note that overeruption of upper 6 has caused some of its root to become exposed. Exposed root decays faster than the crown of a tooth, as we will see later.

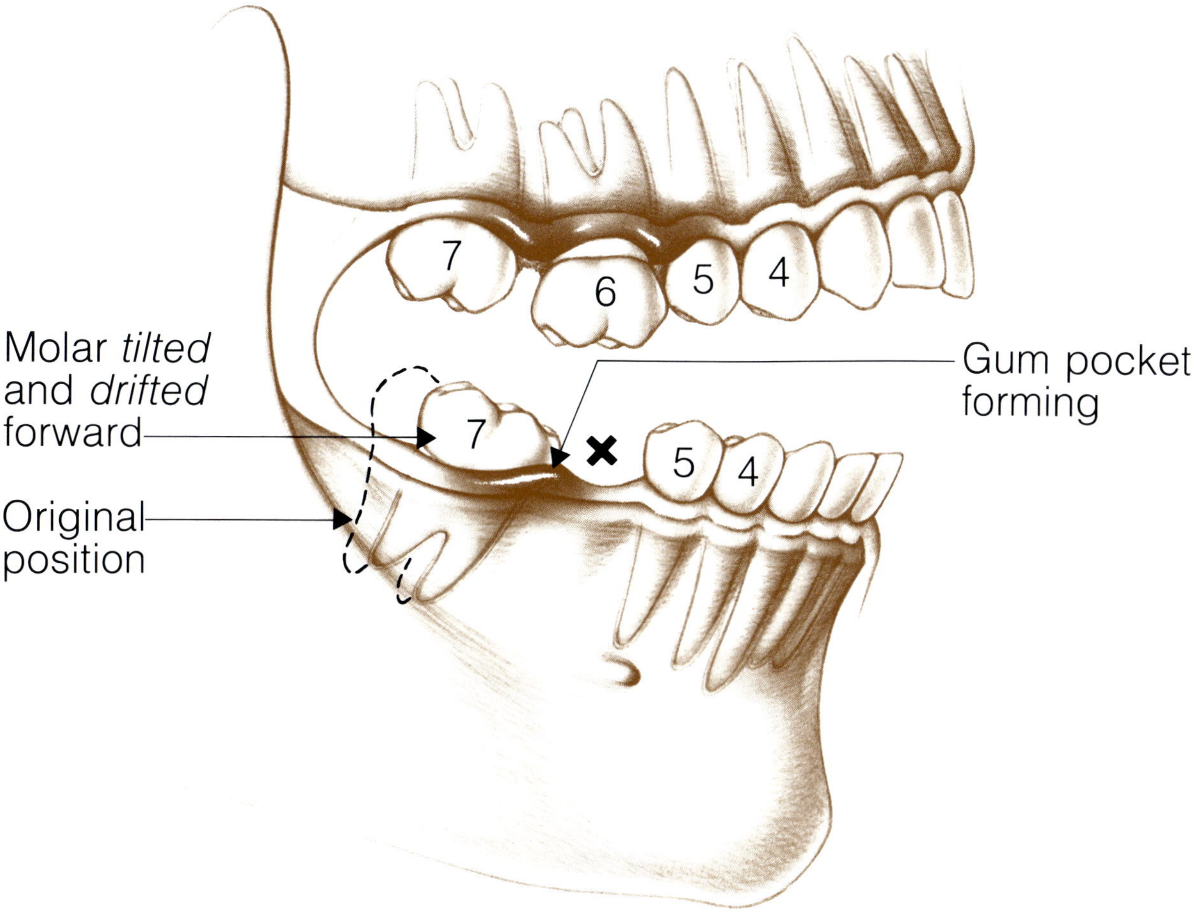

TILT AND DRIFT

Back teeth have a lifetime tendency to *tilt* (lean over) toward the front of the mouth. They also have the potential to *drift* (move) toward the front of the mouth.

Now that a tooth has been extracted from position X, a space is left. This allows lower molar 7 to *tilt* and *drift* forward.

Lower 7 will tilt farther and farther over as you chew on it.

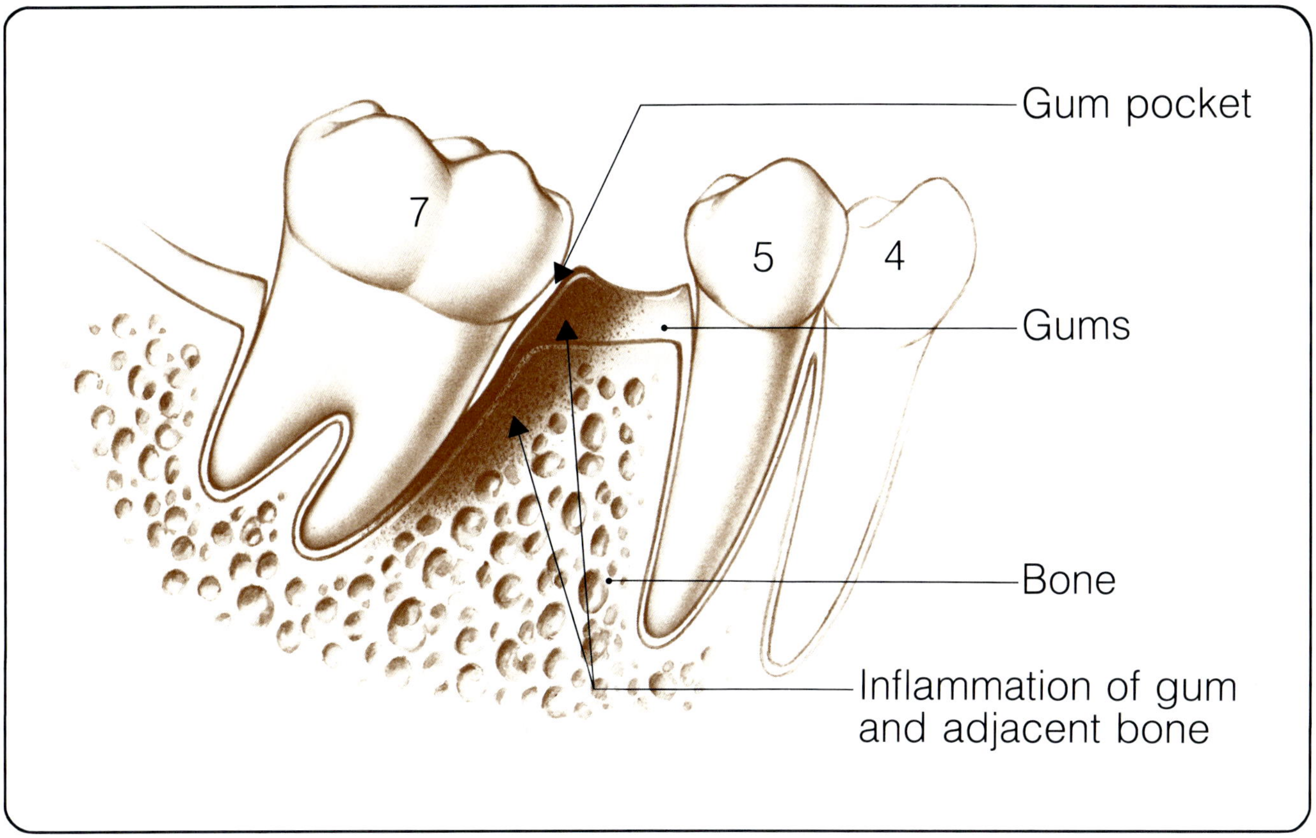

GUM POCKET FORMATION

A tooth tilted over will develop a *gum pocket* along its forward root, as shown here.

Gum pockets are narrow, abnormal spaces or clefts that develop between the gums and the tooth root. These pockets trap food debris and bacteria.

A gum pocket is a problem because you can almost never keep it clean, even with the best brushing and flossing.

The debris and bacteria that collect in a pocket lead to ever-worsening inflammation of the gums adjacent to the pocket.

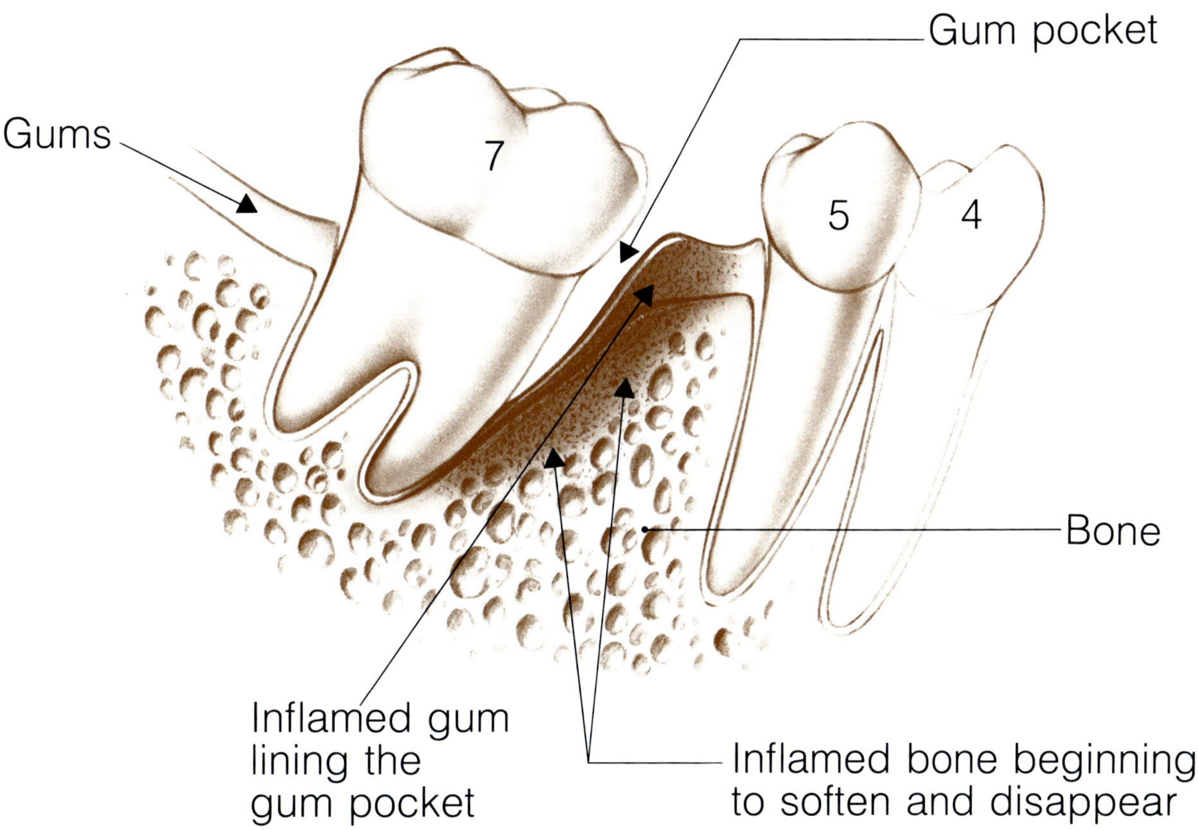

LOSS OF BONE SUPPORTING THE TOOTH

When an area of the gums is constantly inflamed, as you see in this gum pocket, the bone immediately adjacent to it can become inflamed too. *Inflamed bone softens, and slowly begins to disappear.*

This process of gum inflammation and loss of the bone holding a tooth is called *periodontal disease*.*

**This process is shown in* What is Periodontal Disease?, *another booklet in this series.*

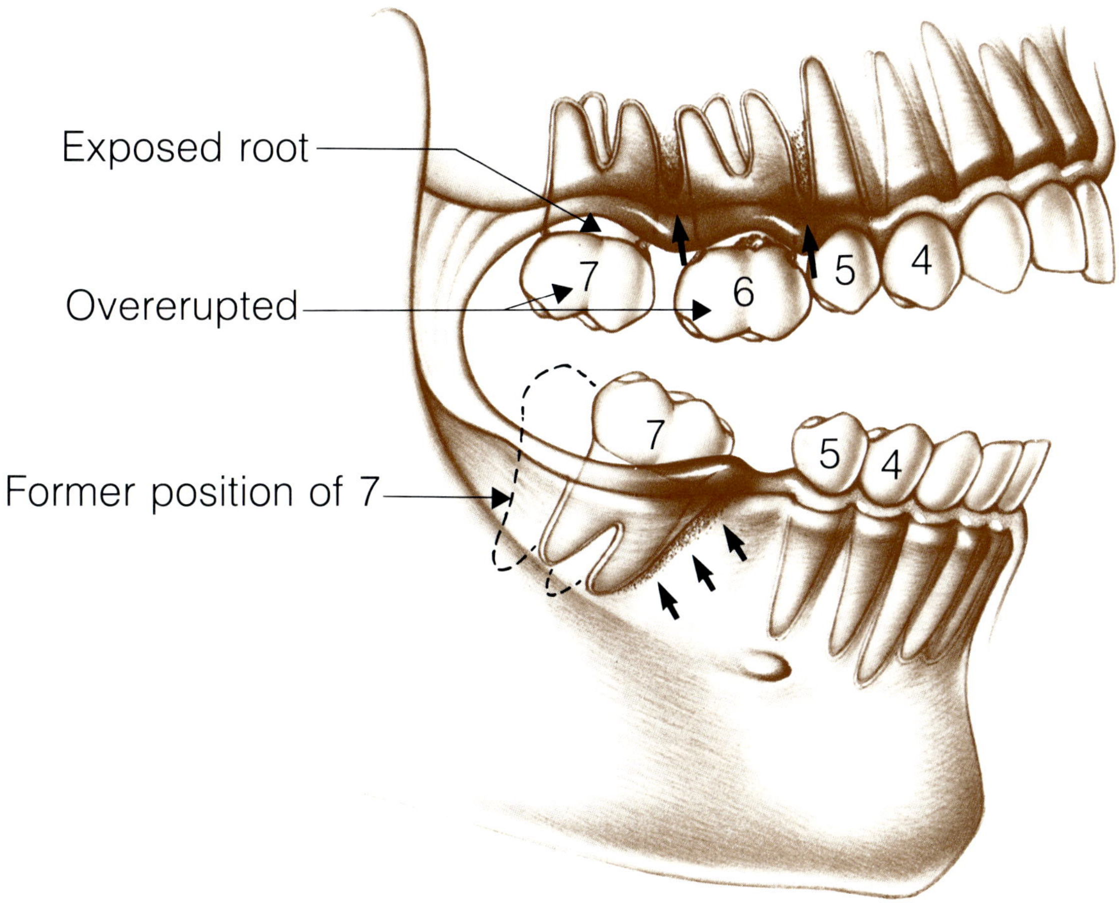

DESTRUCTION SPREADS

Lower molar 7 has drifted and tilted so far forward that upper 7 no longer bites on it. This allows upper 7 to overerupt too. Arrows (↑) show advancing gum pockets, gum inflammation, and bone loss.

Decay has begun on upper teeth 6 and 7, particularly on the exposed portions of the roots of 6 and 7. Exposed roots are especially prone to decay.

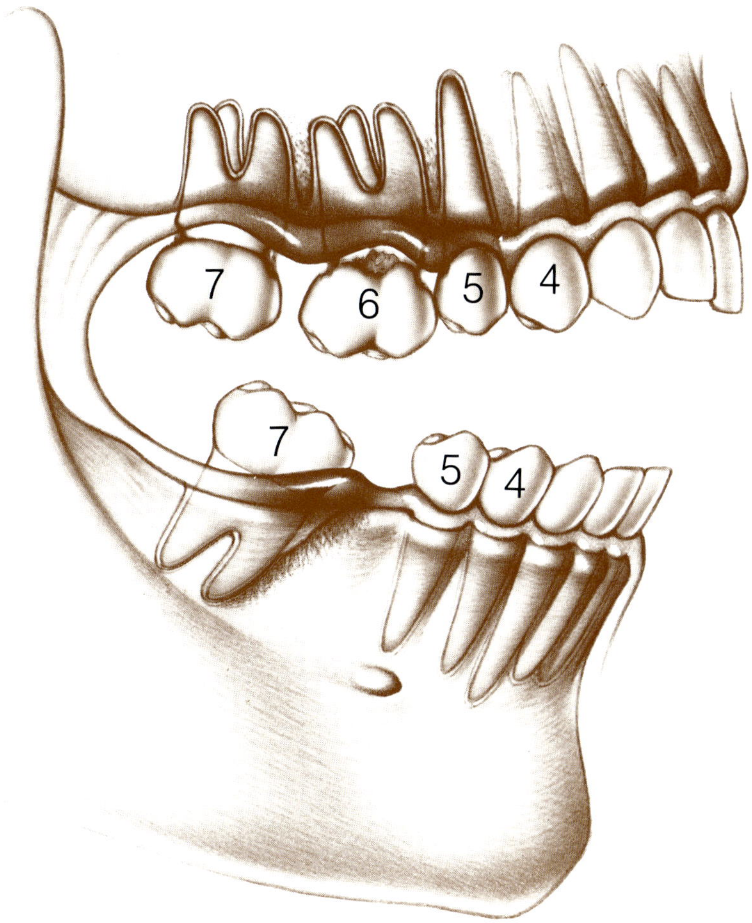

Both upper molars are deeply decayed. Decay has also started on lower 7.

Periodontal disease—gum pockets, gum inflammation, and loss of bone—continues to worsen.

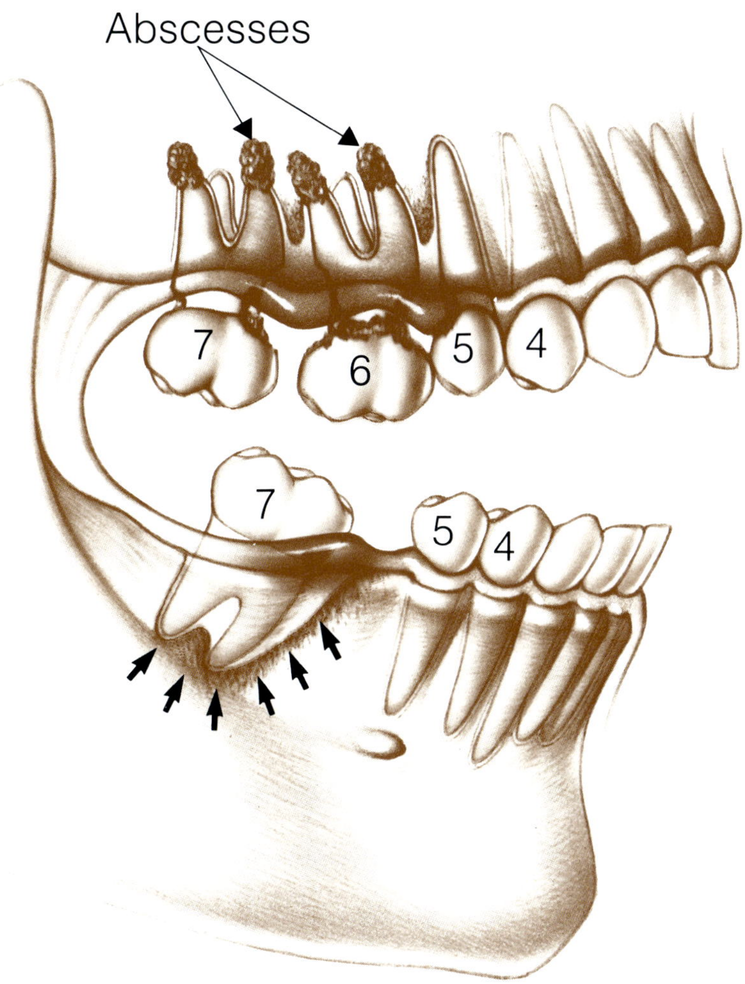

Deep decay has allowed bacteria to enter and infect the *pulps* (''nerves'') of upper 6 and 7. These two teeth have abscessed (become seriously infected). They are so badly damaged by decay that they must be extracted.

Because of inflammation from the gum pocket of lower 7, bone loss (outlined by arrows) has spread around the front root of this tooth and extended to part of the back root too. This tooth has lost so much bone support that it is now loose and must be extracted.

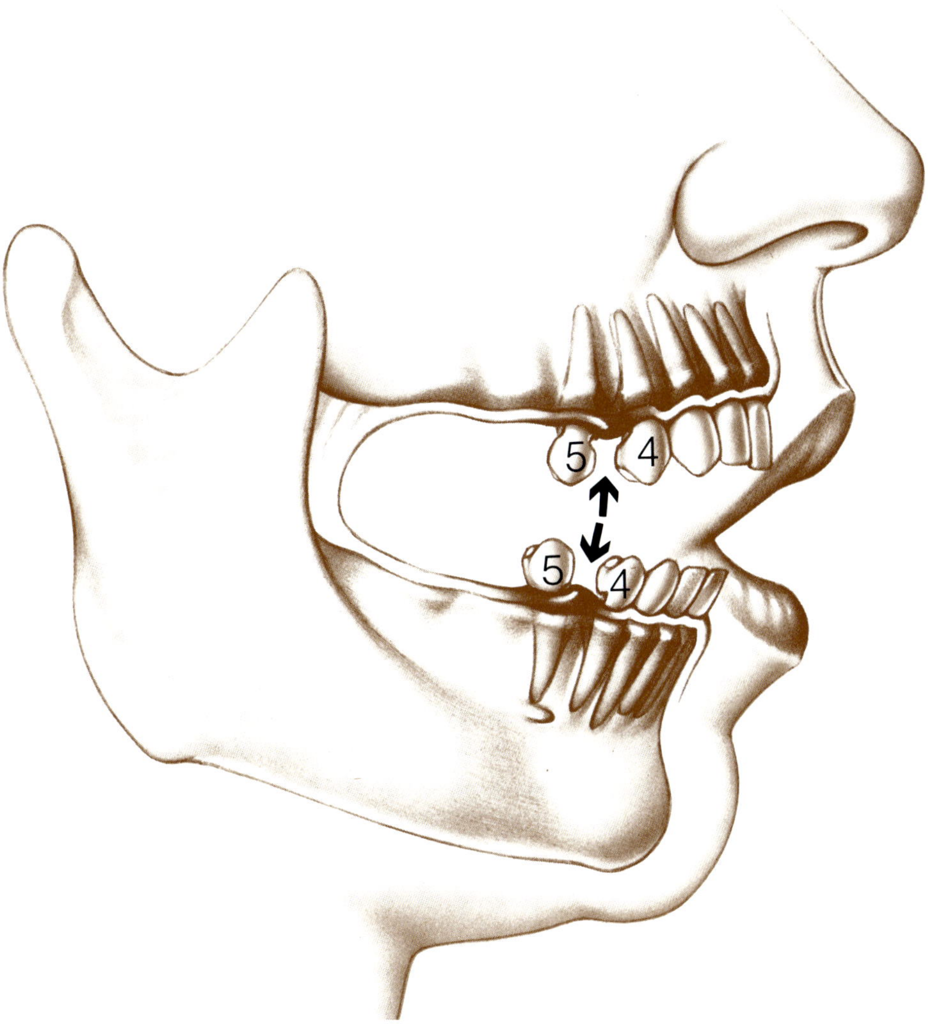

Because all the molars on this side of the mouth have been removed, the upper and lower 5s have no support behind them and are forced backward by the action of chewing.

Food jams between the separated teeth (arrows). Gum inflammation has begun. Gum pockets will follow, along with bone loss and decay. Eventually the 5s will have to be extracted.

After the loss of the upper and lower 5s, the destructive process can move farther forward. The front teeth will start to spread apart, gum pockets will form, decay begin.

Now you may lose your front teeth too.

CONCLUSION

Failure to replace a single molar tooth may start a chain of events: *overeruption, tilt, drift, gum pockets, decay, bone loss.* Over the years this chain of events can lead to the loss of all of your teeth.

Inserting a false tooth today will avoid grief and much greater expense tomorrow.

ISBN 0-86715-135-8

What is Periodontal Disease?

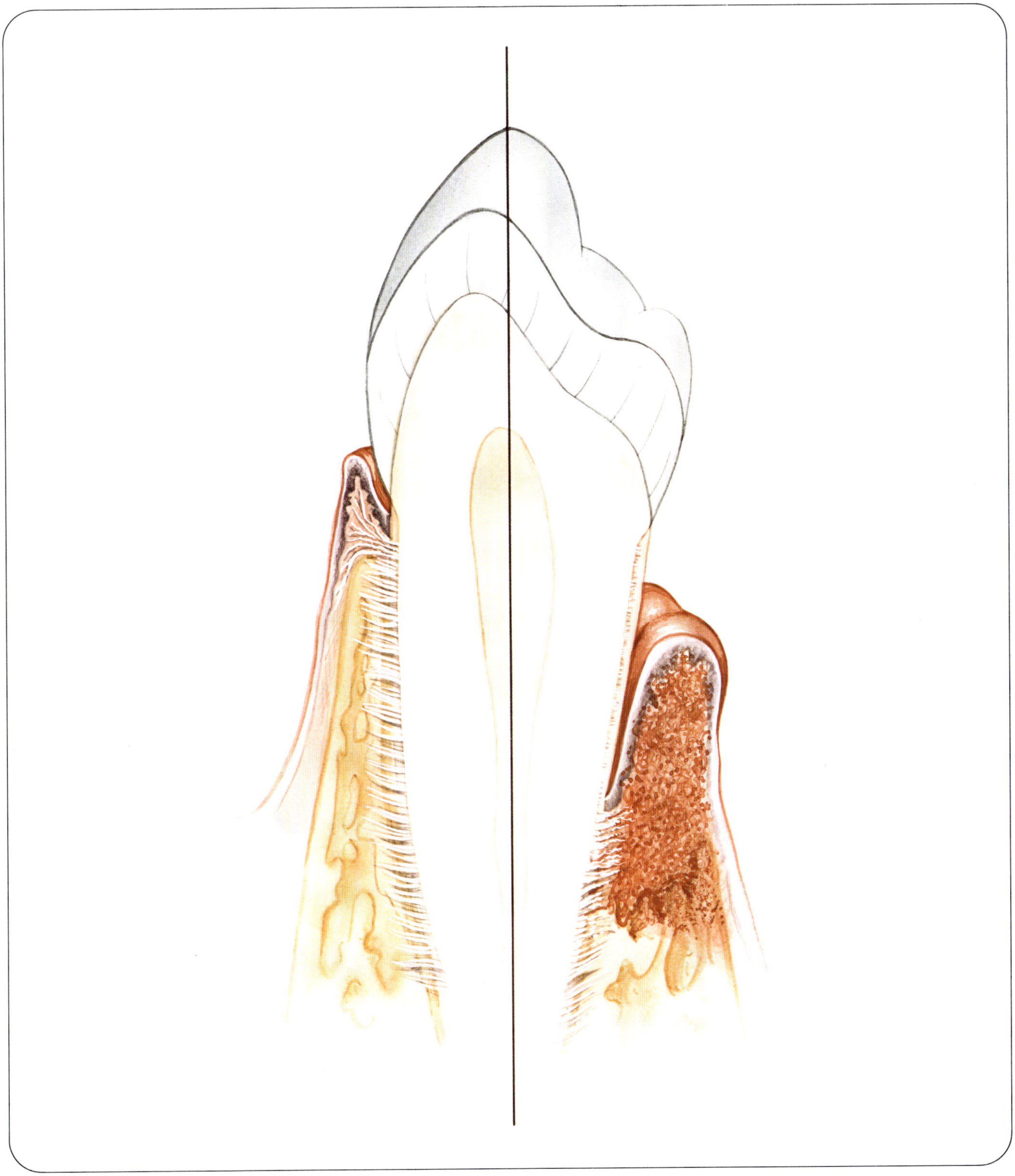

This book is dedicated to the men and women of today who practice modern preventive dentistry, and to their patients who care.

quintessence books

Second Printing, 1984

Art and Text by Explanatory Publications

Artists: Marsha J. Dohrmann and Carol Donner

Lithography: time litho, Leinfelden-Echterdingen
Composition: Bartels & Wernitz, Druckerei und Verlag KG, Berlin
Binding: Schöneberger Buchbinderei, Stiller & Co. KG, Berlin

Printed in Germany

ISBN: 0-86715-109-9

Periodontal disease affects four out of every five people. It can start very early in life. It causes the loss of more teeth than all other reasons combined.

What is periodontal disease? Who gets it?

How does it start? Can you prevent it?

Can it be successfully treated once it has started?

This booklet answers these questions.

This publication explains general principles. There are individual exceptions. Your own dentist's advice is the best advice you can get.

PART I

PART I gives you general information about periodontal disease: its signs, its cause, and what you and your dentist can do to slow down or prevent the disease.

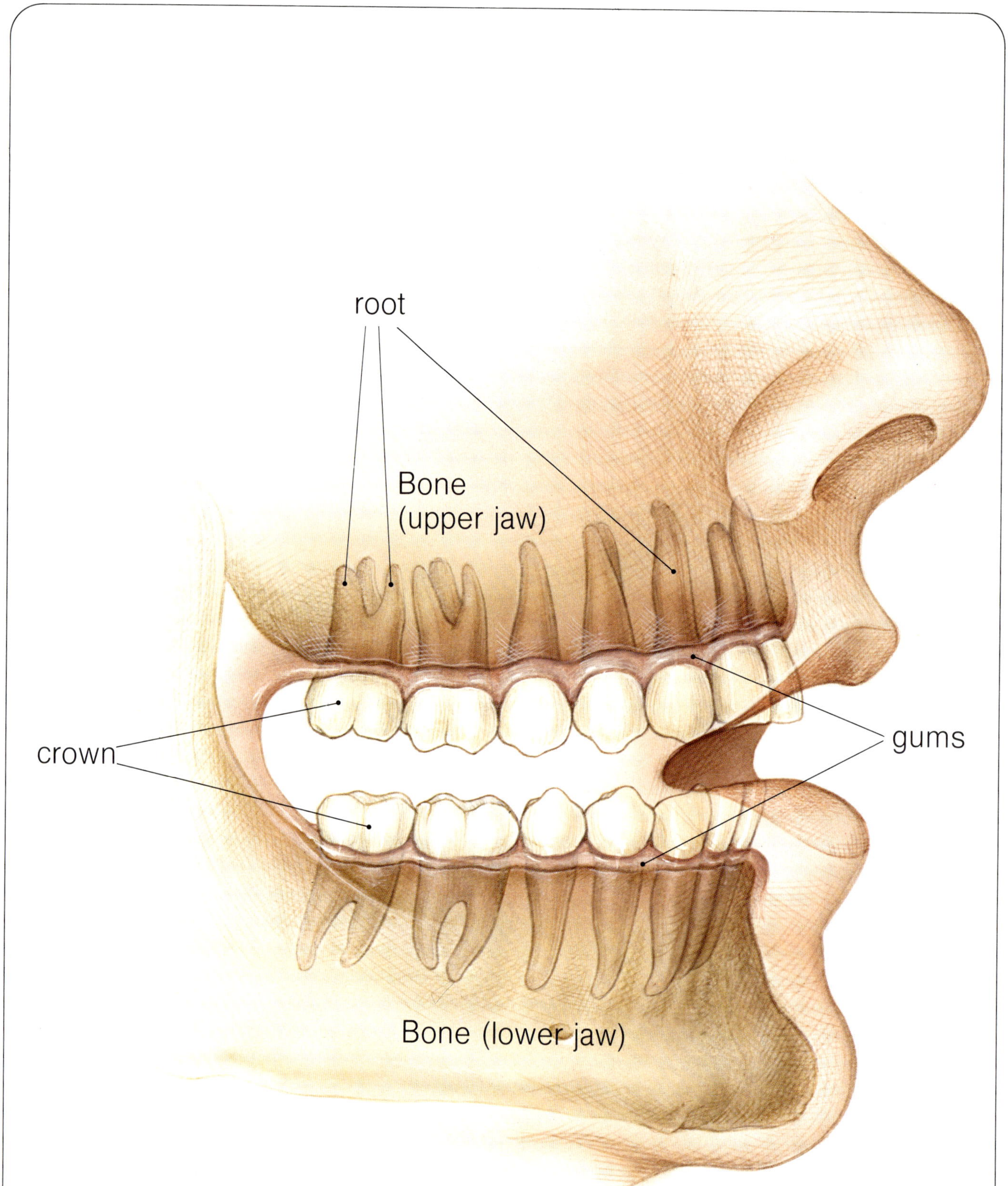
root
Bone
(upper jaw)
crown
gums
Bone (lower jaw)

INTRODUCTION

Each tooth consists of two parts: the *crown* and the *root(s)*.

Only the crown is visible in the mouth. The roots are in the bone.

The *neck* of the tooth is where the root(s) and crown meet.

The *gums* are a protective type of skin that clings to the necks of the teeth and covers the bone holding the teeth.

Some teeth have one root, others have two or three roots.

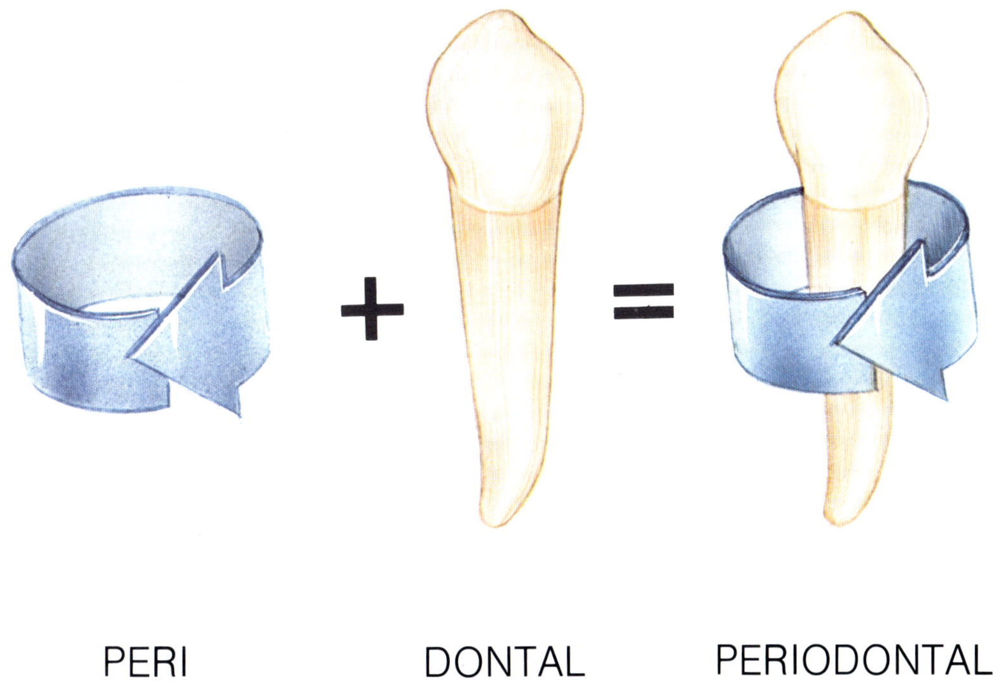

Peri means "around".

Dontal means "tooth".

Periodontal means "around-the-tooth."

Periodontal disease ("around-the-tooth disease") attacks the *gums* around the teeth, and the *bone* that supports the teeth.

NORMAL GUMS

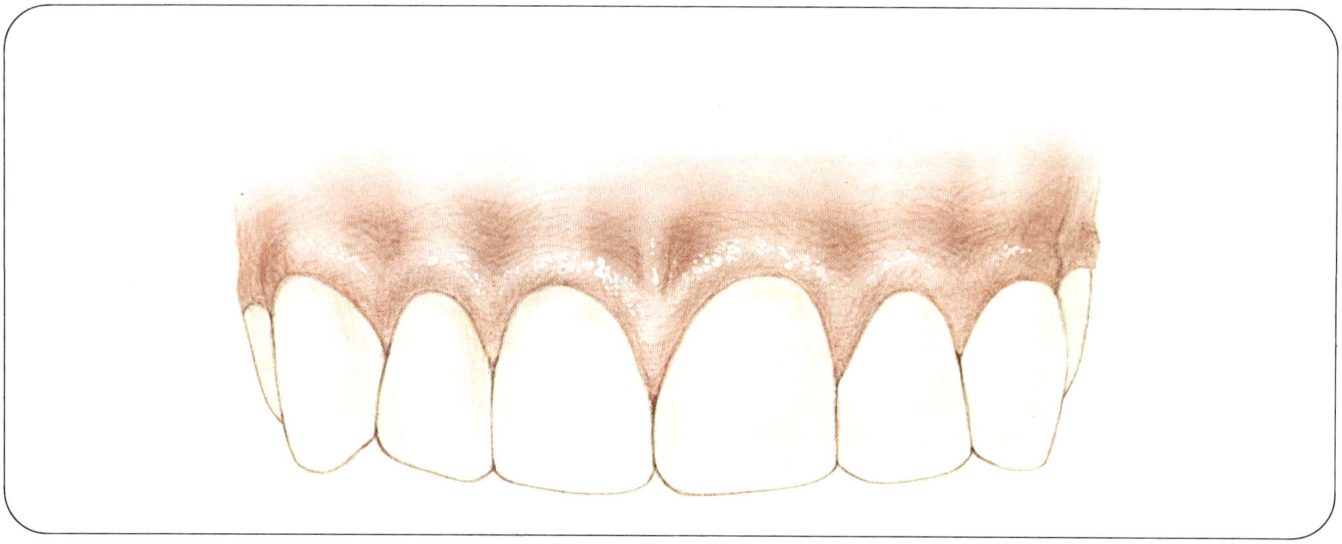

This diagram shows the gums of a person who has a light complexion. People with dark skin have gums normally quite a bit darker.

SEVEN SIGNS OF PERIODONTAL DISEASE

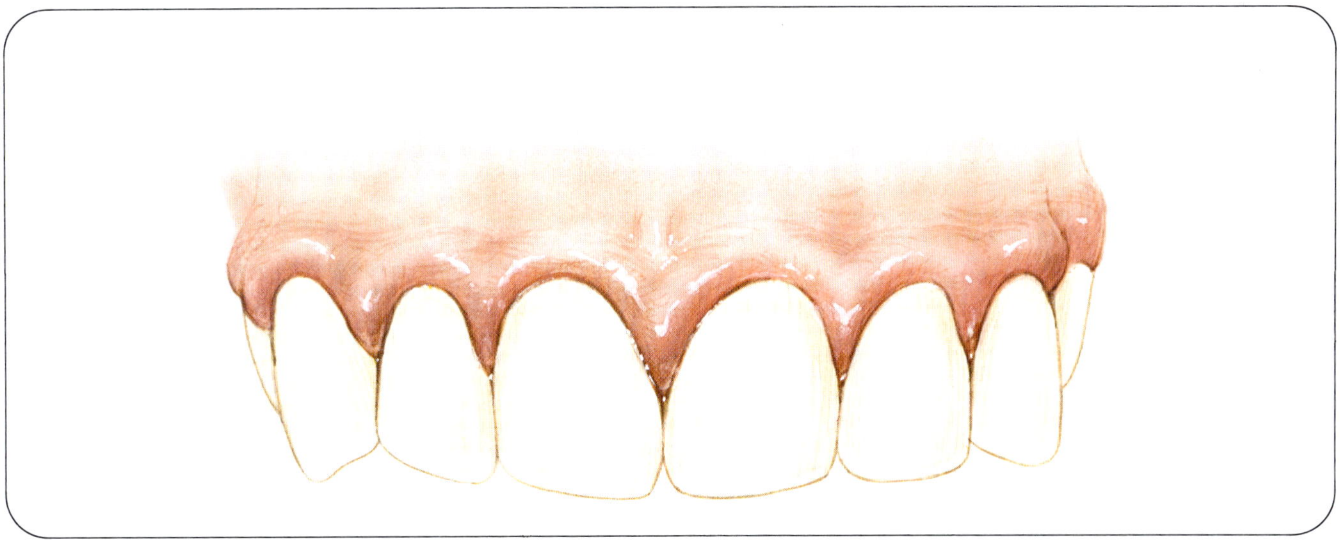

1. *Gums red and puffy*. No matter what a person's complexion, gums should never be red or swollen like those shown above.

2. *Bleeding gums*. Gums should never bleed, even when you brush vigorously or use dental floss. *If your gums bleed, even sometimes, something is wrong*.

3. *Persistent bad breath*. Bad breath can be a sign of periodontal disease. You may not notice it yourself. Your family can help by telling you.

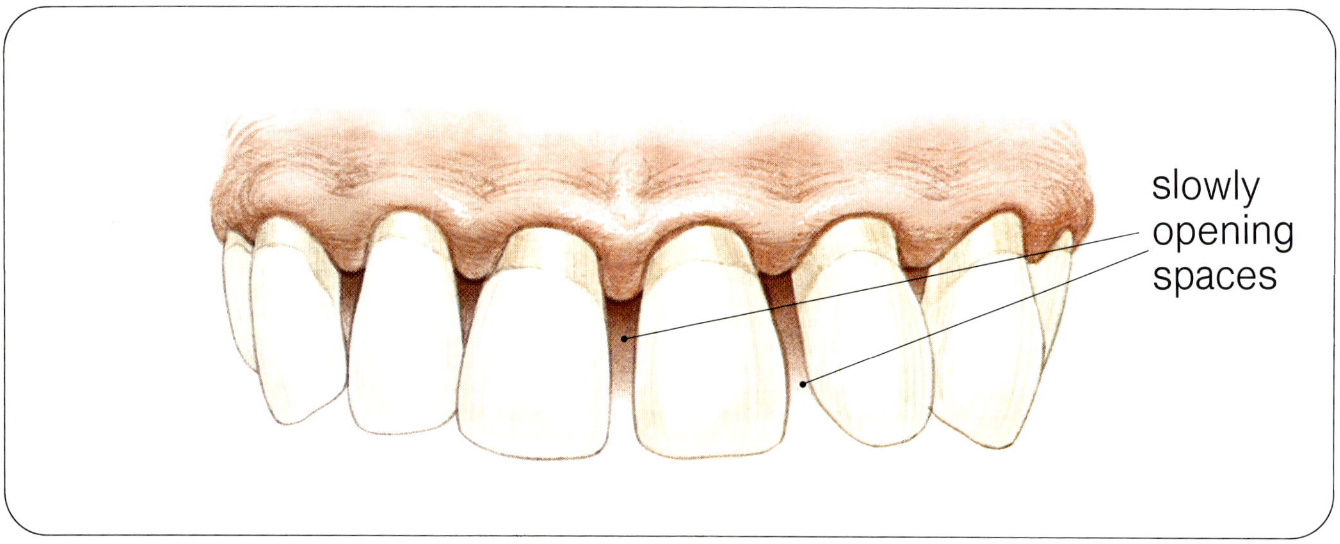

4. *Spaces that begin to appear between the teeth.*

5. *One or more teeth begin to loosen.*

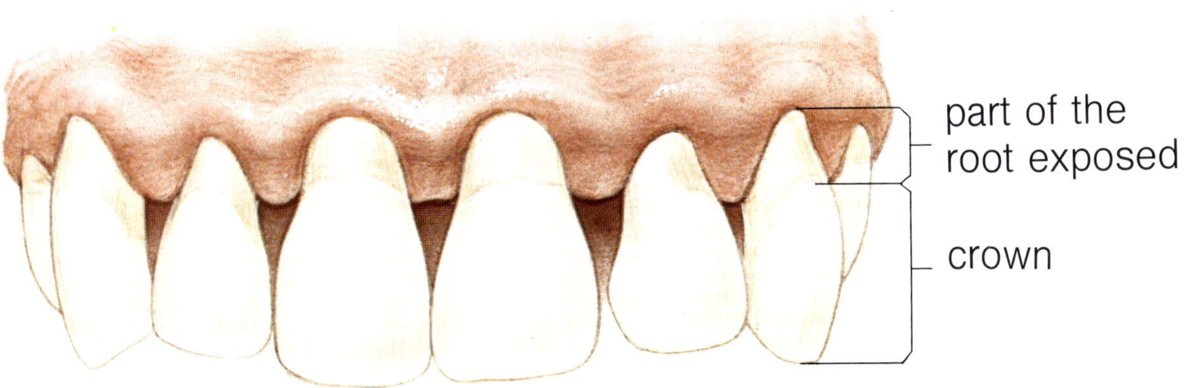

6. *Receding gums*. Disease causes the gums to shrink away from the crown, and expose some of the root. This makes the teeth look longer.

People of *advanced* age may have minor receding not caused by periodontal disease. But, any receding at any age should make you suspicious until your dentist says it is normal for you.

7. *Vague aching or itching or other discomfort*.

Periodontal disease is almost always *painless* in the early stages. Therefore, you may not notice the gradual onset of puffiness of your gums, or pay attention to occasional bleeding when brushing. Or you may think the longer look of your teeth is normal for your age. *Four out of five teenagers and adults have periodontal disease, and most don't know it*. That is why people lose more teeth from periodontal disease than from all other reasons combined.

But the good news is that *most periodontal disease can be prevented*; or if already started, *it can be treated*. This is particularly true *if it is recognized in its early stages*.

PLAQUE IS THE CAUSE OF PERIODONTAL DISEASE

Every day a sticky, almost invisible film forms on the teeth. This film is *plaque**. It is a growing colony of living bacteria. Plaque also contains a little food debris and saliva.

In very large amounts plaque can be seen, particularly at the gum line.

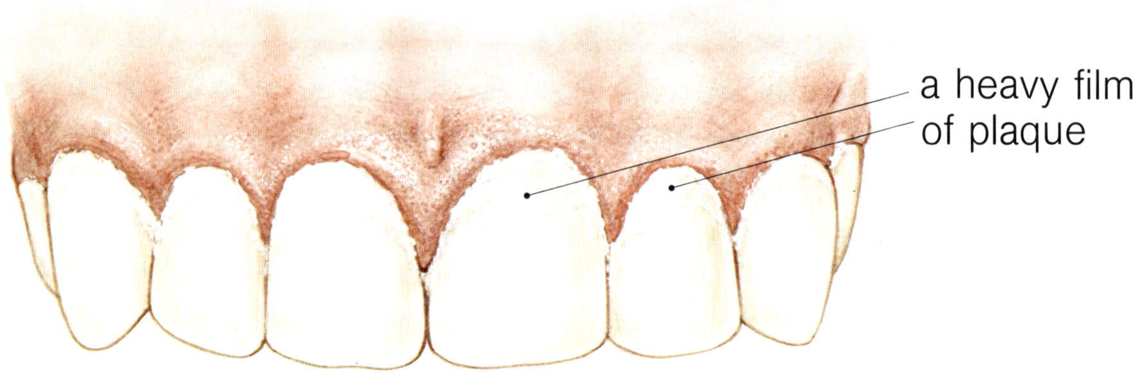

In large amounts plaque can be felt with the tongue as a fuzzy, unclean coating on the teeth.

*pronounced "plack"

The bacteria of plaque produce *toxins* (poisons) that inflame the gums.

This inflammation is the start of periodontal disease!

PLAQUE BECOMES CALCULUS

If you do not completely remove plaque every day by toothbrushing and flossing, it leads to the formation of *calculus* ("tartar"), a stony crust with a pitted, rough surface.

It takes only a little over a day for any plaque you leave on your teeth to turn into calculus.

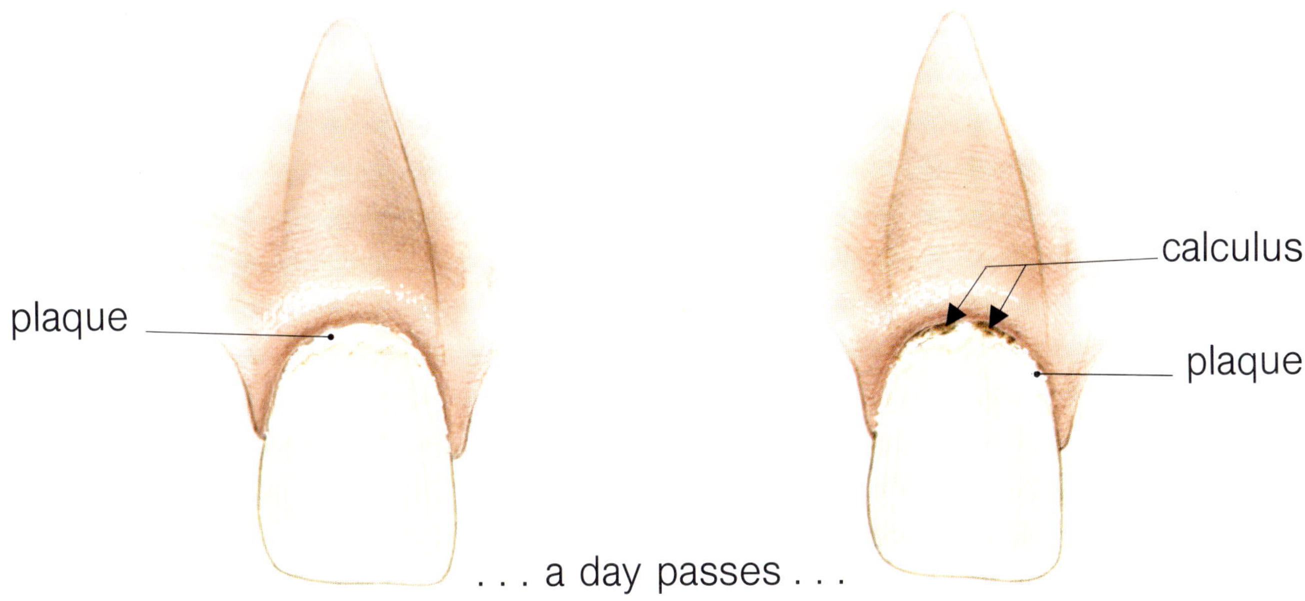

Plaque you should have removed by brushing or flossing from the smooth surface of the tooth.

Plaque that you left has now become *calculus* which you cannot remove yourself.

You can't remove calculus yourself. It clings to the teeth with such force that only a dentist or hygienist can remove it.

It is possible to see calculus that forms *above* the gums. It appears as a brownish or black deposit around the necks of the teeth. However, *it is the hidden calculus under the gums* that does the most harm.

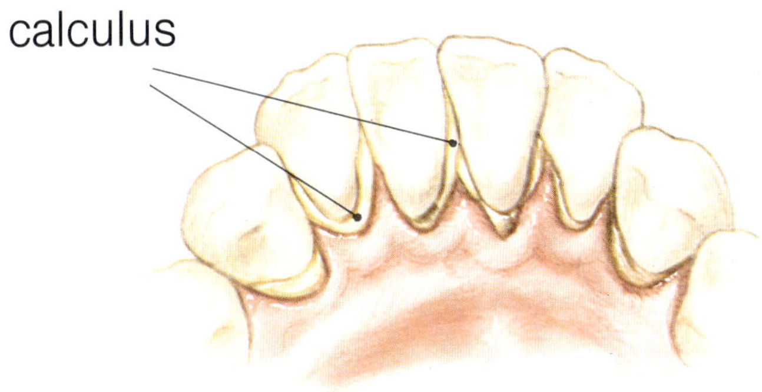

Backs of lower front teeth, just in front of the tongue, a common place to see calculus build-up.

Calculus greatly complicates the problem of preventing periodontal disease. Each day's new plaque embeds itself in the rough surface of calculus in such a way that *no toothbrush or dental floss or any other home dental device can ever remove it*!

Thus, all calculus will always have plaque embedded on its surface. And all plaque is capable of starting or worsening periodontal disease.

Obviously, it is very important never to let calculus get a start. Brush and floss away plaque every day. Never let plaque remain long enough to become calculus.

Miss brushing and flossing for one day and you can give first calculus its start.

To sum up:

YOU CAN remove sticky plaque from your teeth.

YOU CAN'T remove calculus yourself, or remove the plaque that forms on the surface of any calculus.

PLAQUE TOXINS DESTROY BONE

The toxins produced by the bacteria of plaque not only inflame the gum, but also *cause destruction of the bone* just underneath.

As the gum inflammation continues, the bone destruction continues too, usually without any symptoms in the early stages of the disease.

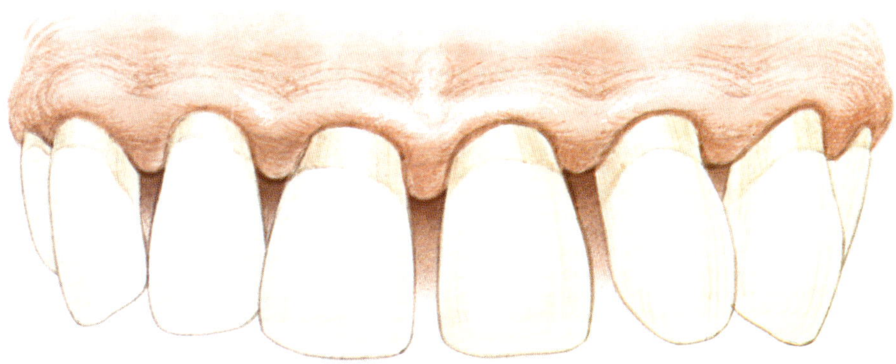

ADVANCED PERIODONTAL DISEASE

Disease has caused severe receding of the gums, and has destroyed half the bone holding these teeth. These teeth are loose.

When sufficient bone has been lost, the tooth loosens. When a tooth loosens, the destruction of bone around it accelerates.

Finally, when deprived of most of its supporting bone, the tooth becomes so loose it either falls out or must be extracted.

NATURAL RESISTANCE OR SUSCEPTIBILITY TO PERIODONTAL DISEASE

A few people are very *resistant* to periodontal disease. Some are highly *susceptible*.

However, most people have a varying resistance to the disease at different times in their lives. For example, a person's resistance may be normal for years. Then, for no apparent reason, resistance temporarily diminishes. Periodontal disease then appears; or, disease that was under control flares up.

No one knows why resistance varies from person to person, or why it varies in the same person at different times. Dental research teams around the world are searching for answers.

But, no matter what your susceptibility or resistance, you and your dentist together can slow down, or check this disease. For the vast majority of people, loss of all the teeth to periodontal disease is *not* inevitable.

PREVENTION

To prevent or treat any periodontal disease *you and your dentist must work together*:

WHAT YOU MUST DO

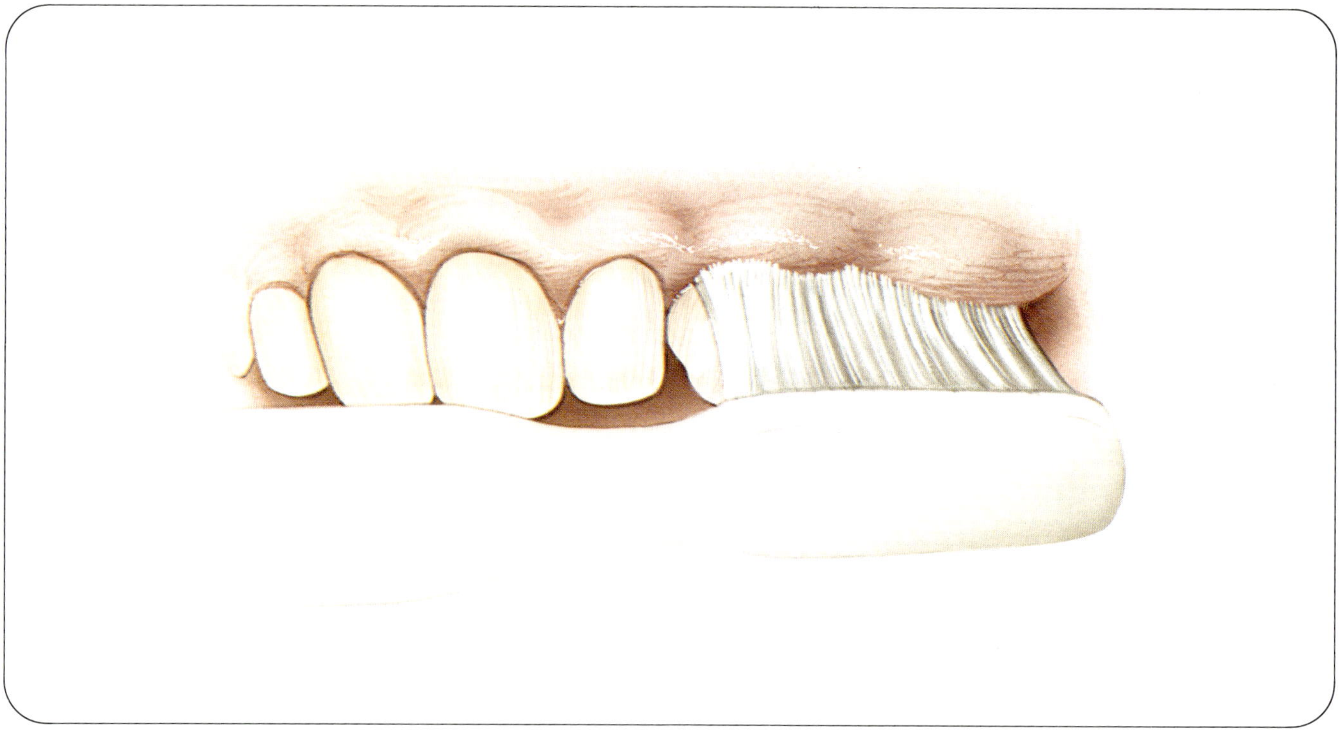

You must *brush correctly* every day.

Toothbrush bristles remove the plaque from exposed surfaces of the teeth.

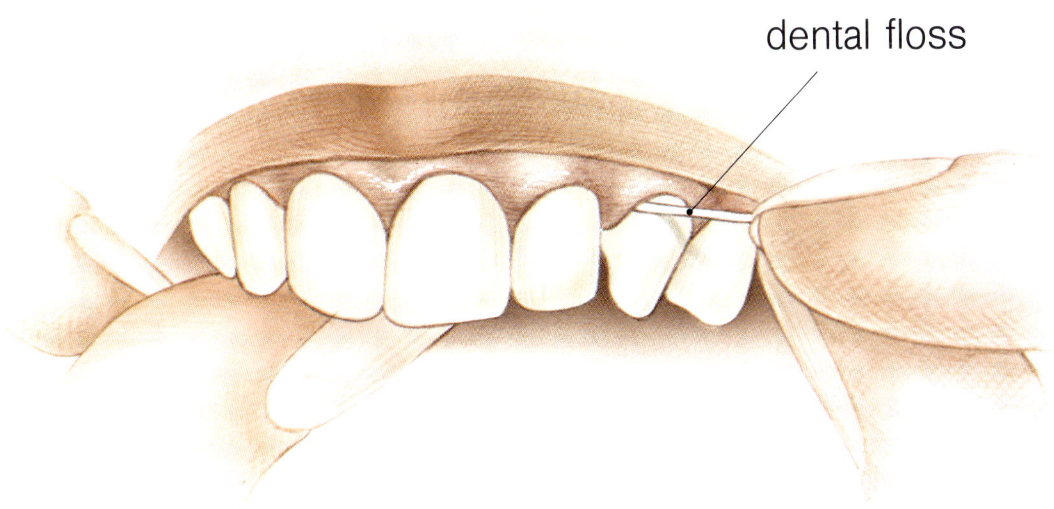

You must *floss correctly* every day.

Dental floss removes the plaque from between the teeth where bristles can't reach.

If you brush but don't floss, you are doing only *half* the job, and there is little your dentist can do to help you.

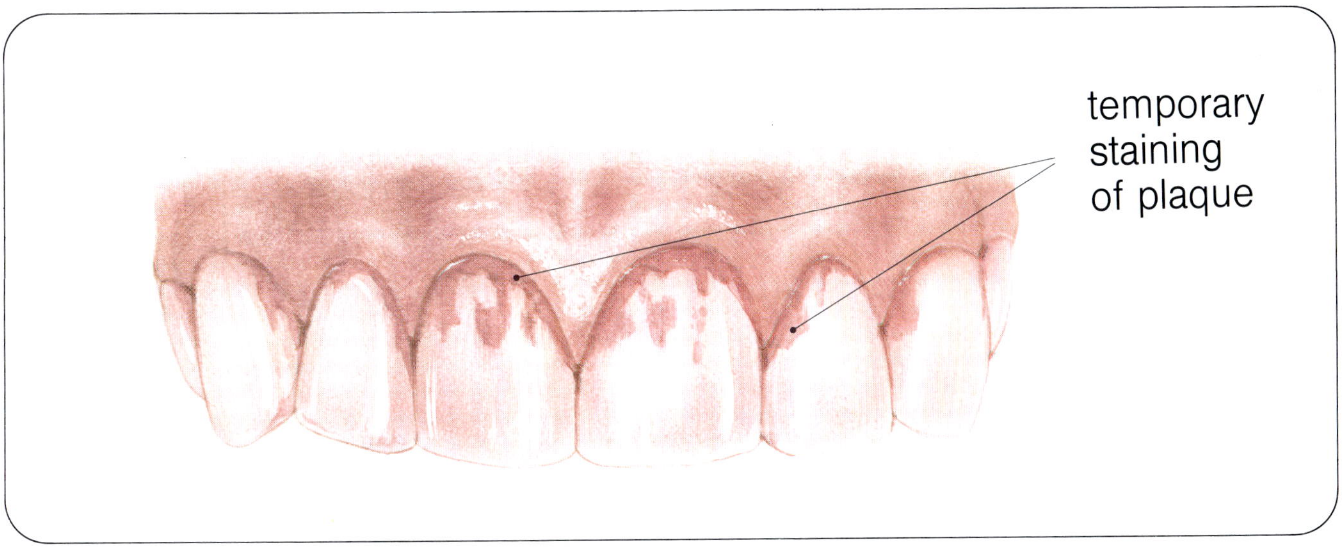

Drugstores sell inexpensive *disclosing tablets* that contain a harmless vegetable dye. You should occasionally dissolve one in your mouth after brushing and flossing. It will temporarily stain any plaque you have missed, showing you areas you must make a special effort to clean more thoroughly.

WHAT YOUR DENTIST CAN DO

Don't depend upon diagnosing early periodontal disease yourself. It may start between back teeth where you can't see it; it will almost always be painless; and, in the beginning, there may be no "pink toothbrush" (bleeding) to warn you.

Therefore, even if you never have cavities, and your mouth feels fine, *go for regular dental check-ups*. Your dentist and hygienist can spot early disease, when it is the easiest – and least costly – to treat.

Your dentist will note the color of your gums, look for swollen gums, and check for loosening teeth.

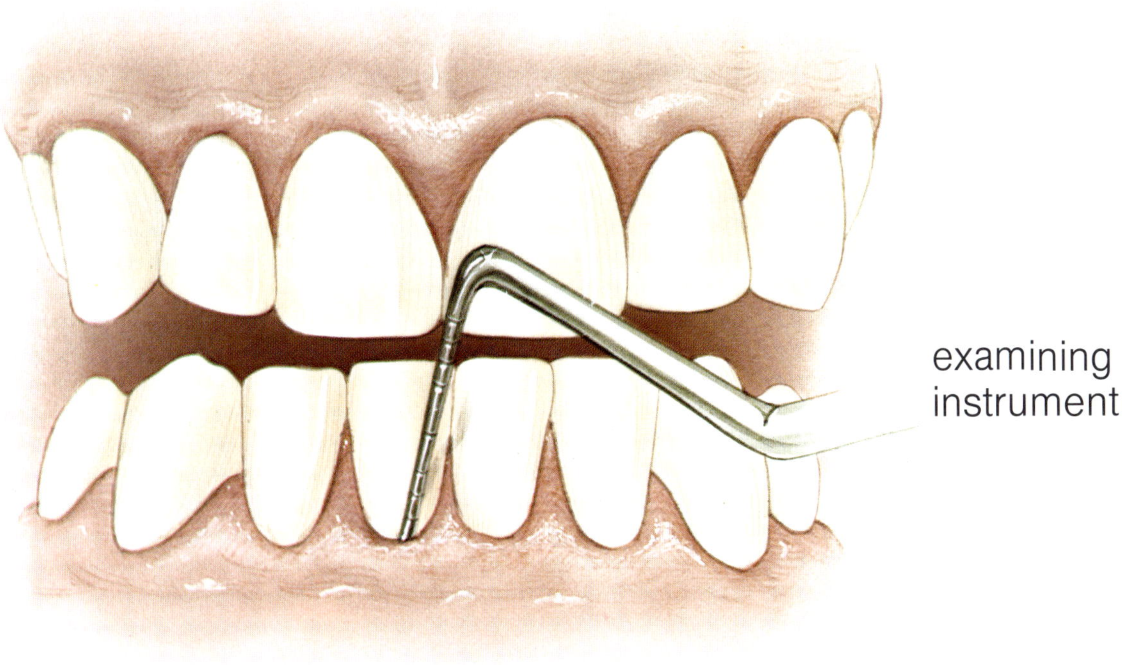

He will gently examine all the gum crevices for hidden areas of disease.

He may review your diet with you to be sure you are getting proper nutrition.

Note:
Although the pronoun "he" appears, it refers to men *and* women dentists.

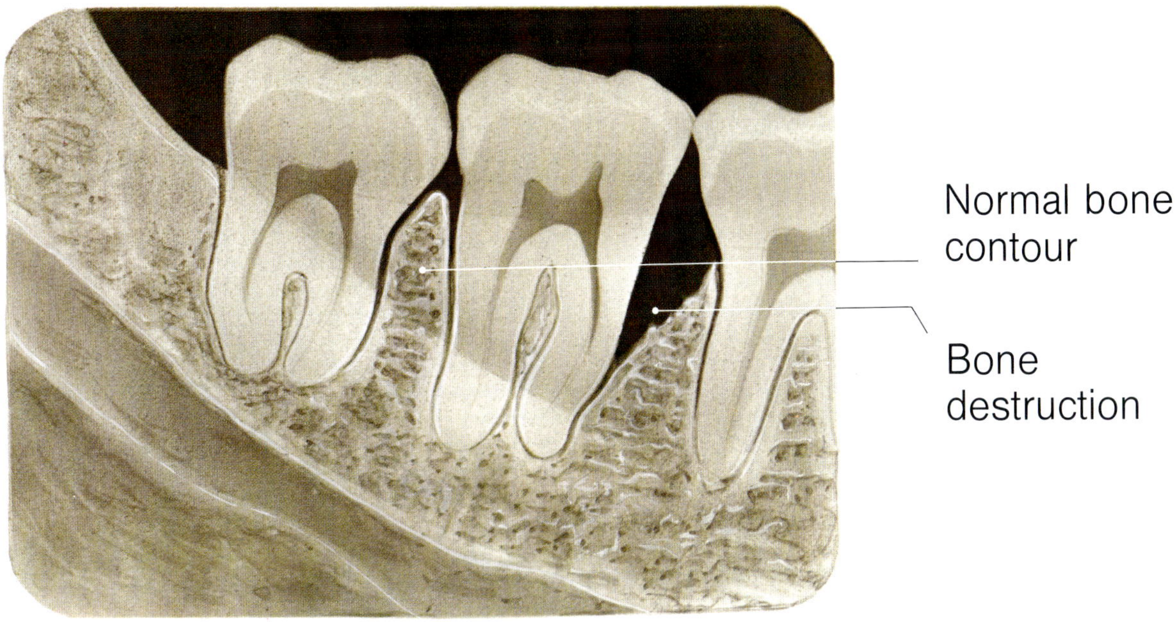

X-ray

He will take X-rays to look for bone destruction in its *early* stages.

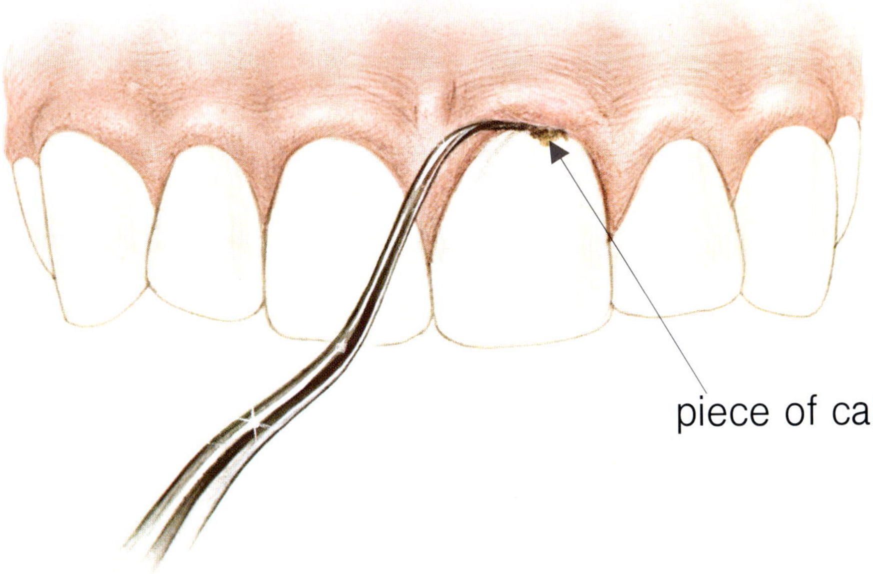

Despite the best home care, some calculus may form. Your dentist or the hygienist will gently remove it.

Your dentist will check any *gold or porcelain dental crowns* as well as any *dental fillings* for *correct shape and fit*. Fillings and crowns that no longer fit precisely may cause severe periodontal problems. He will repair or replace them.

Your dentist will inspect the way your upper and lower teeth come together (the "bite") to see if the forces of chewing are evenly distributed among all the teeth. If you are chewing on some teeth harder than others, he will gently reshape the biting surfaces of these teeth until they meet evenly.

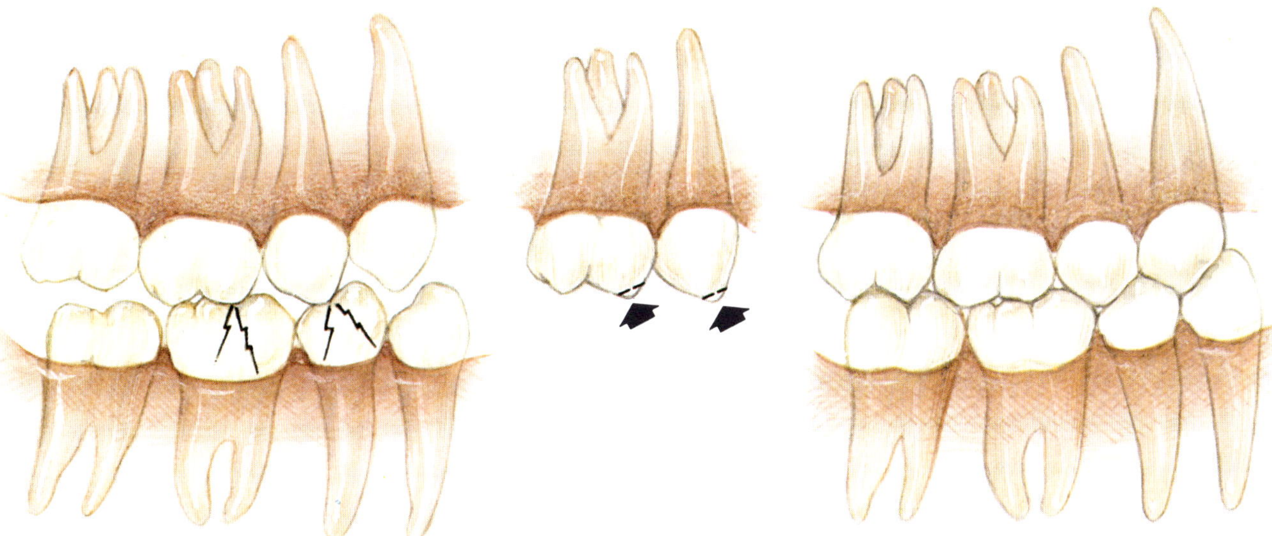

A

Before reshaping: points on two of the upper teeth hit hard on the lowers.

B

The points will be polished down to the dotted lines.

C

A *balanced bite*: all the teeth meet evenly.

A *balanced bite* (one where the teeth meet evenly during chewing) is important for many reasons, but it is crucial when periodontal inflammation is being treated. Too much force on a tooth with periodontal disease causes bone loss to happen faster.

One of the most important things a dentist or his trained staff will do is *take the time to teach you proper brushing and flossing*. Few people do it correctly without instruction. The fee you should expect to pay for this valuable service is the best bargain in dentistry. The cost of *not* learning to brush and floss the right way could be the loss of your teeth.

THE SPECIALIST

If you have a periodontal problem that does not respond to routine care, your dentist may refer you to a *periodontist*.

A periodontist is a specialist in the care of the gums and supporting bone. He has years of extra schooling and experience that permit him to use special techniques to treat more difficult or more advanced periodontal problems.

CONCLUSIONS OF PART I

Plaque, a sticky colony of living bacteria, causes periodontal disease.

If you don't brush and floss the *plaque* away every day, it may become a stony crust on the teeth called *calculus*.

Any calculus that forms will permanently embed plaque on its rough surface. This plaque remains stuck to the calculus no matter how well you brush and floss.

Toxins of any plaque can inflame the gums and destroy tooth-supporting bone.

When periodontal disease destroys all the bone holding the tooth, the tooth falls out or must be extracted.

Seven signs of periodontal disease are:

Bleeding gums. *Your gums should never bleed*!
Puffy, red gums.
Spaces beginning between the teeth.
Longer looking teeth.
Constant bad breath.
Teeth loosening.
Vague aching or itching in the gums.

See your dentist on a regular basis, even if you think nothing is wrong. Only a professional can diagnose periodontal disease in its earliest stages when it is the easiest – and least costly – to treat. Loss of all your teeth from periodontal disease is *not* inevitable. You and your dentist, working together, can see to that.

PART II

PART II will tell you how, step by step, periodontal disease causes the loss of a tooth.

First, some important relationships between the teeth, the gums, and the bone.

The teeth within the square below will appear in all the diagrams that follow.

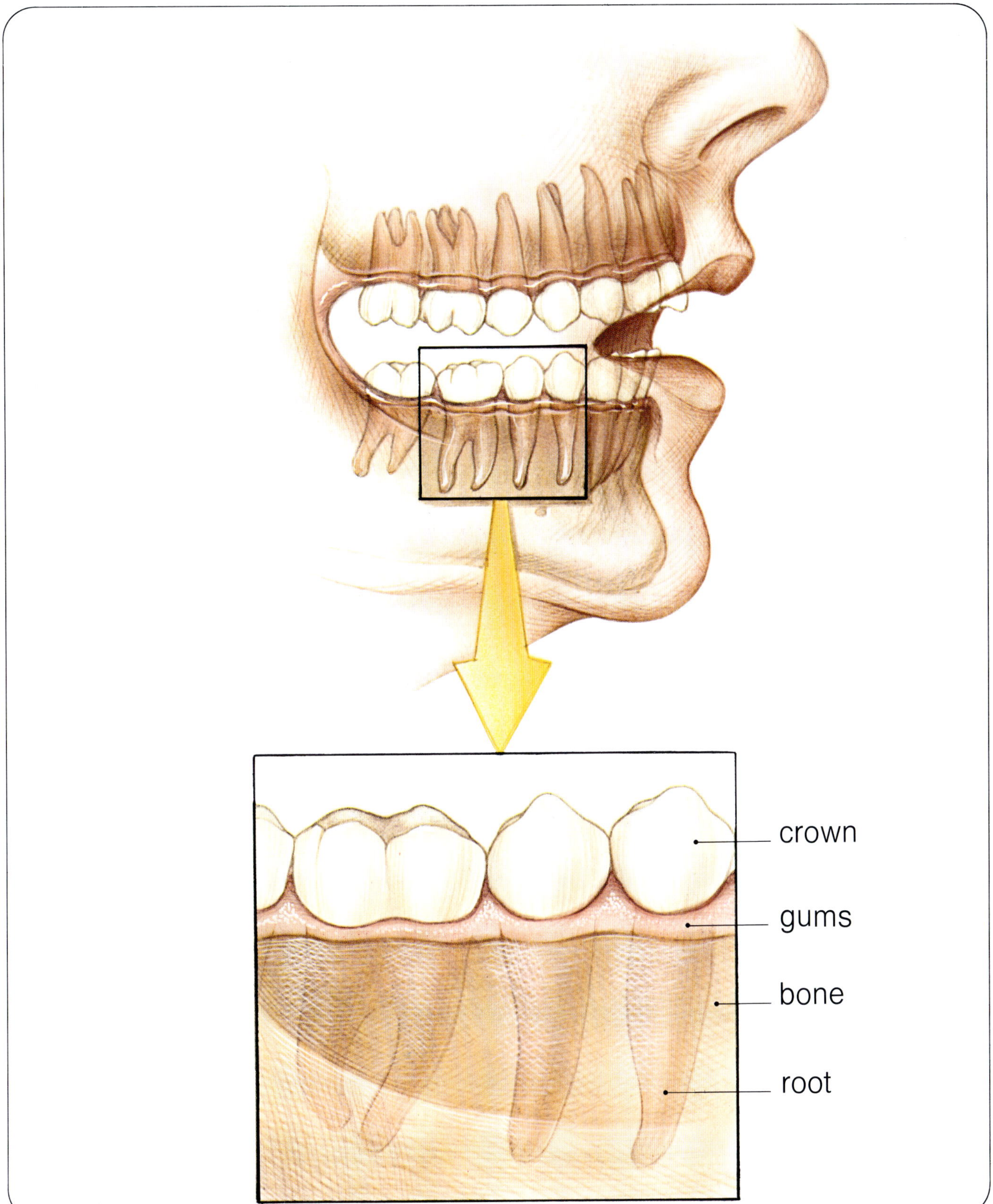

The next drawing shows what is beneath the surface.

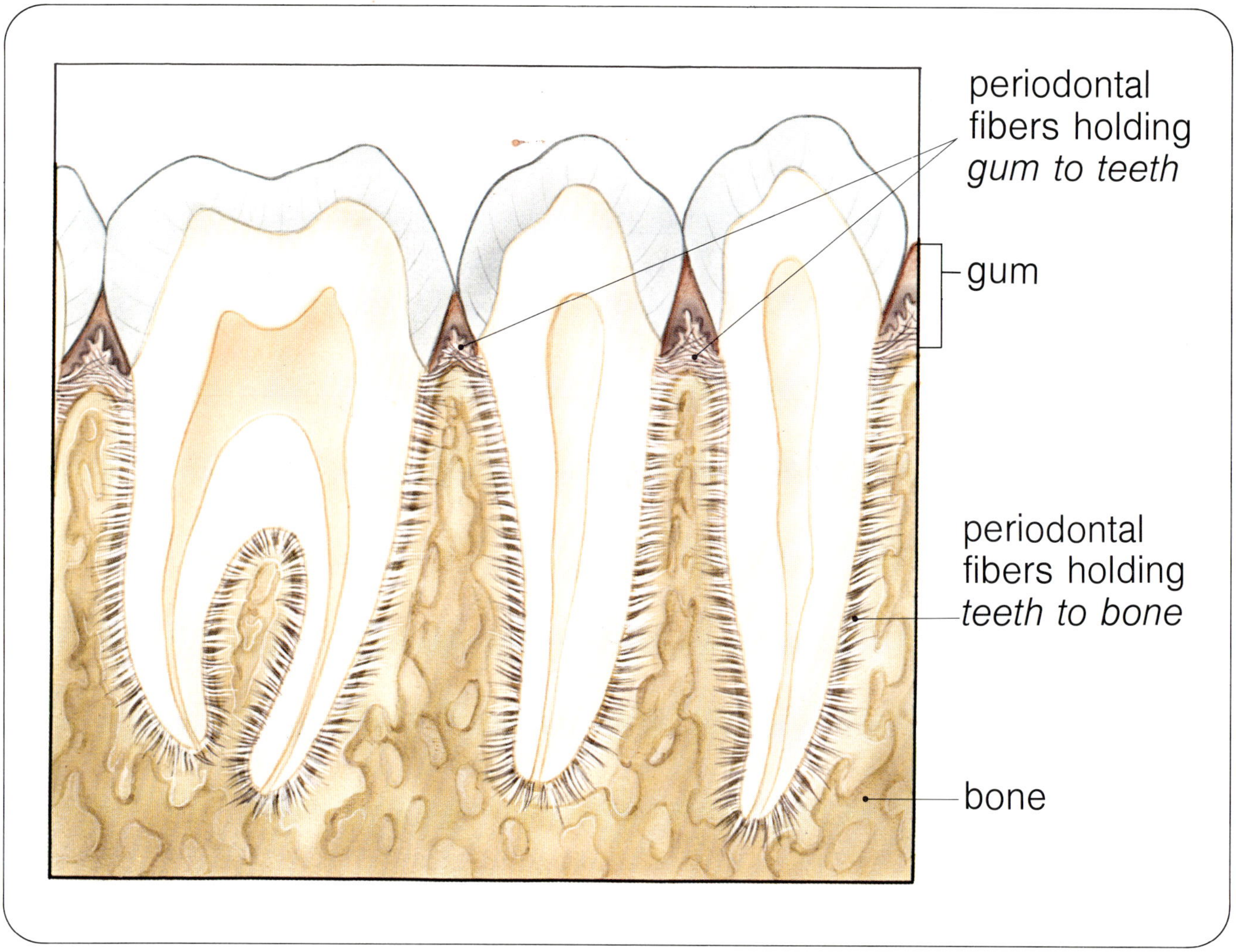

Many thousands of fibers, called *periodontal fibers*, go from their origins on the roots of the teeth into the gums, or into the surrounding bone.

Those *fibers that enter the gums* pull the gums into a tight collar around the necks of the teeth.

The great mass of *fibers that go from the roots into the bone* attach the teeth to the bone.

Some people mistakenly conceive of teeth being "in the gums". Not so. Teeth are in bone. The gums are a protective covering over this bone. In a healthy mouth, the gums hug the teeth like tight collars to prevent bacteria and food debris from invading the bone. Simply put, the gums protect the bone, and the bone holds the teeth.

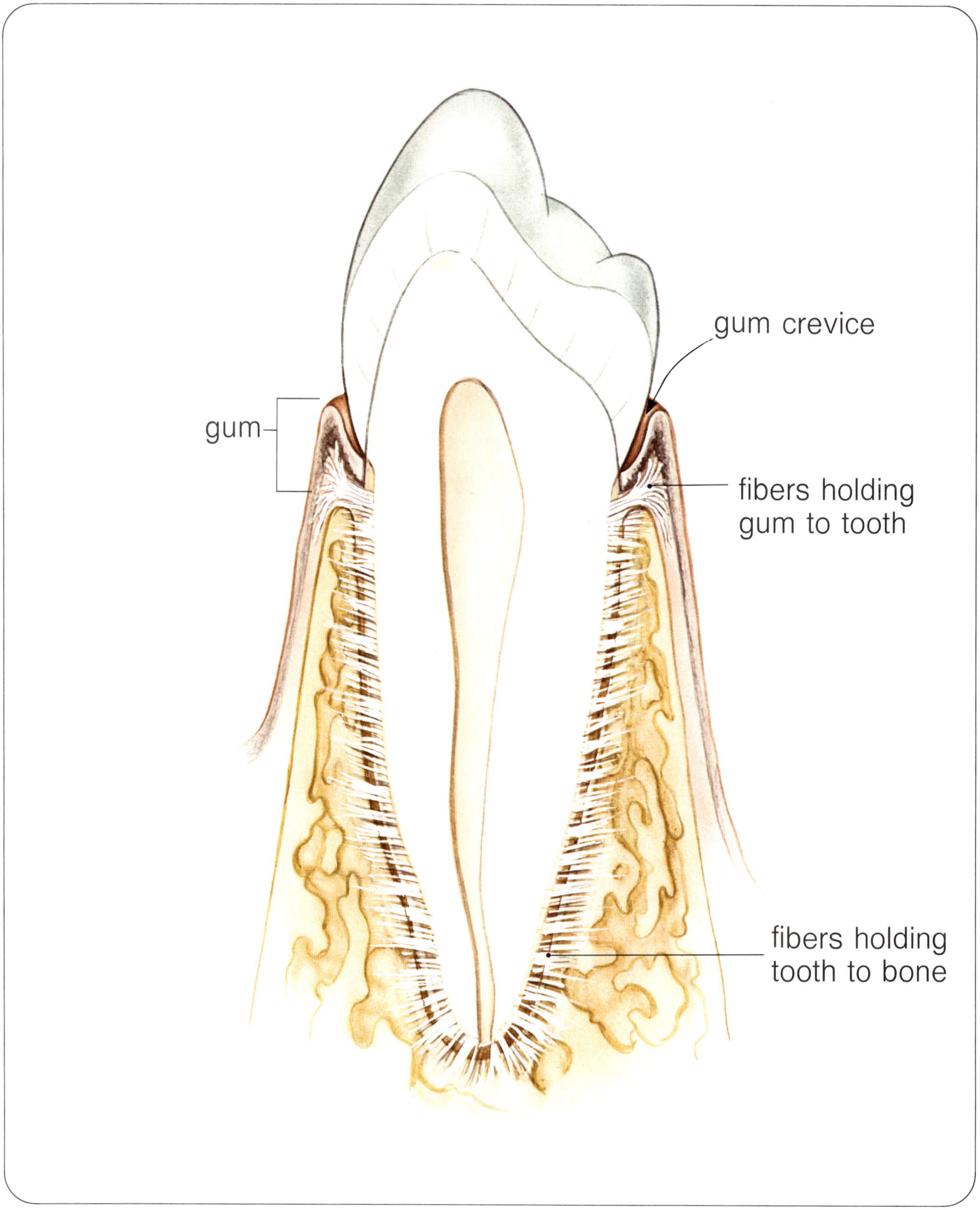

This isolated tooth is enlarged nine times the normal size.

The fibers going from the root into the gum pull the gum tightly against the crown. This is the reason you don't see an actual space between the gum and the crown when you look in the mouth.

This area, where the gum lies against the crown, has been called the *gum crevice*.

We shall see that the depth of this crevice is of major importance.

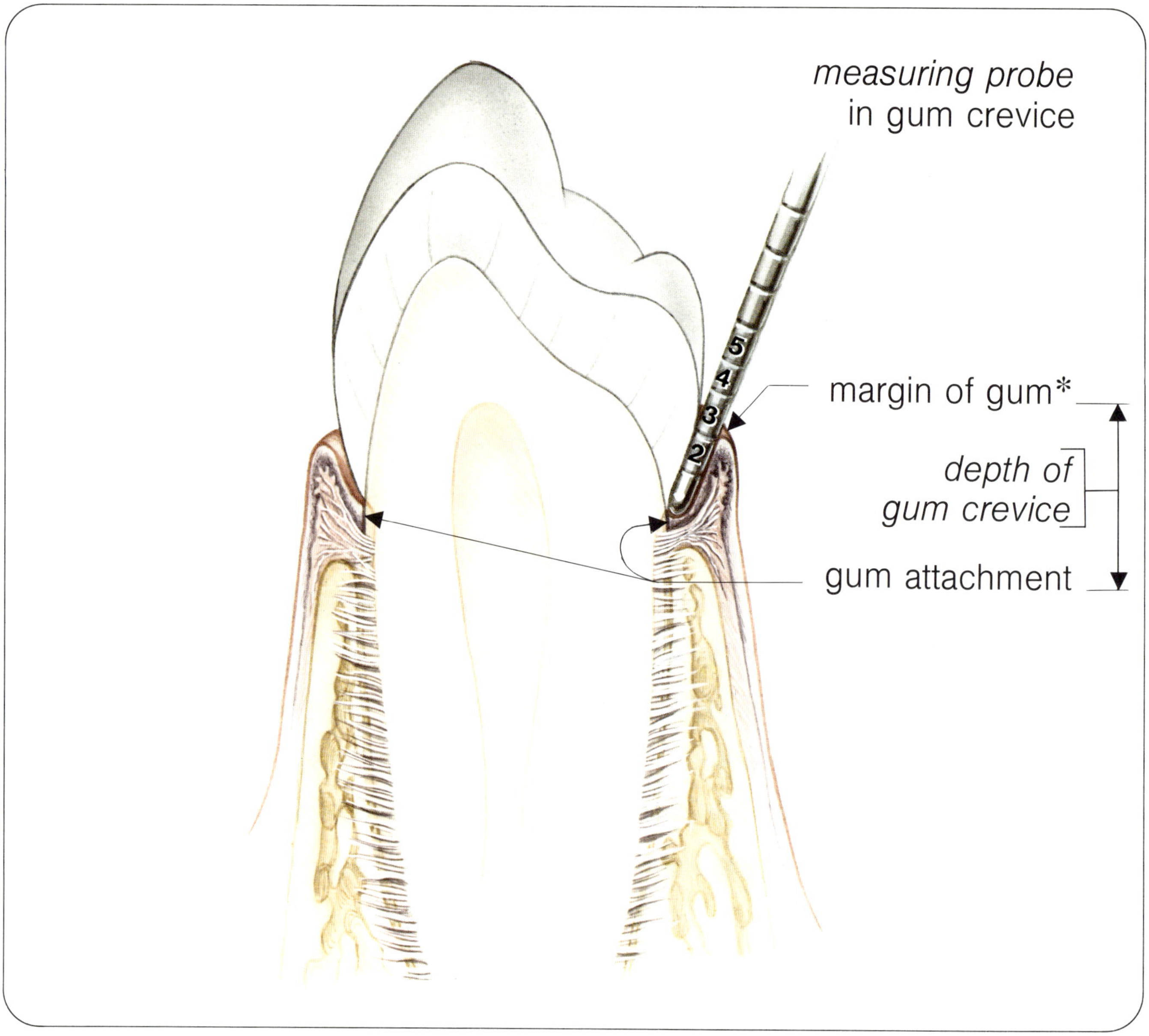

We have placed a dental measuring instrument gently to the bottom of the crevice to measure how deep it is. The *attachment of the gum* limits how far the instrument can go.

*The *margin* of the gum is its upper edge.

The markings on the instrument, called a *periodontal probe*, are one millimeter apart. (An actual millimeter is the distance between these two lines =.)

Normal crevices measure *1 to 3 millimeters* deep. This crevice is 2 millimeters in depth.

Now you have the information you need to understand how periodontal disease actually progresses. To simplify, we have divided the disease into *five different stages*. But, in reality, it is *one continual process*.

Keep in mind as you read that *you and your dentist can prevent periodontal disease*. And, even if it has started, *you and your dentist together can treat it*. This beginning-to-end process need not happen. Loss of your teeth is *not* inevitable.

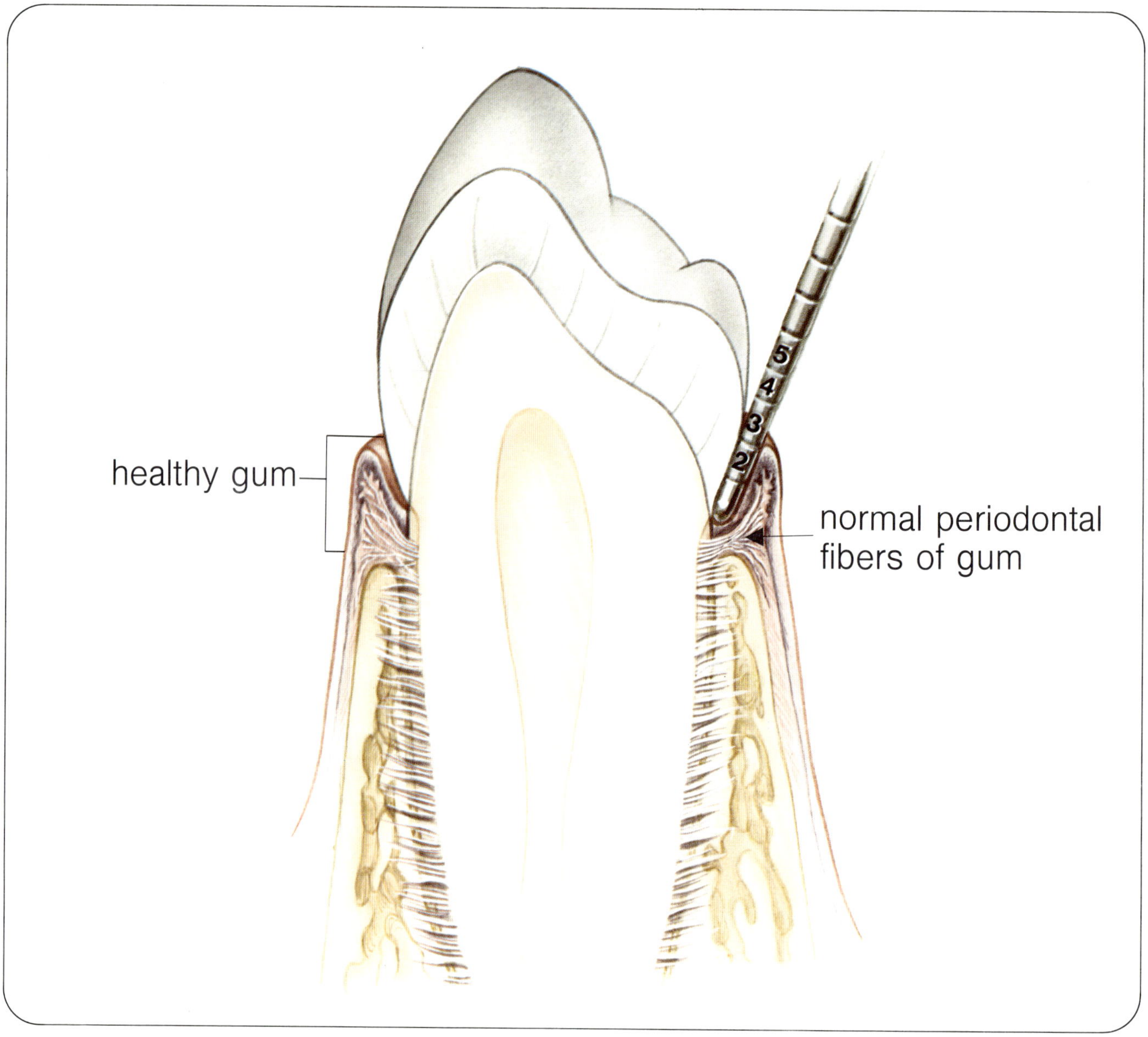

THE NORMAL

Periodontal fibers hold the normal, pink
gum tightly against the tooth.

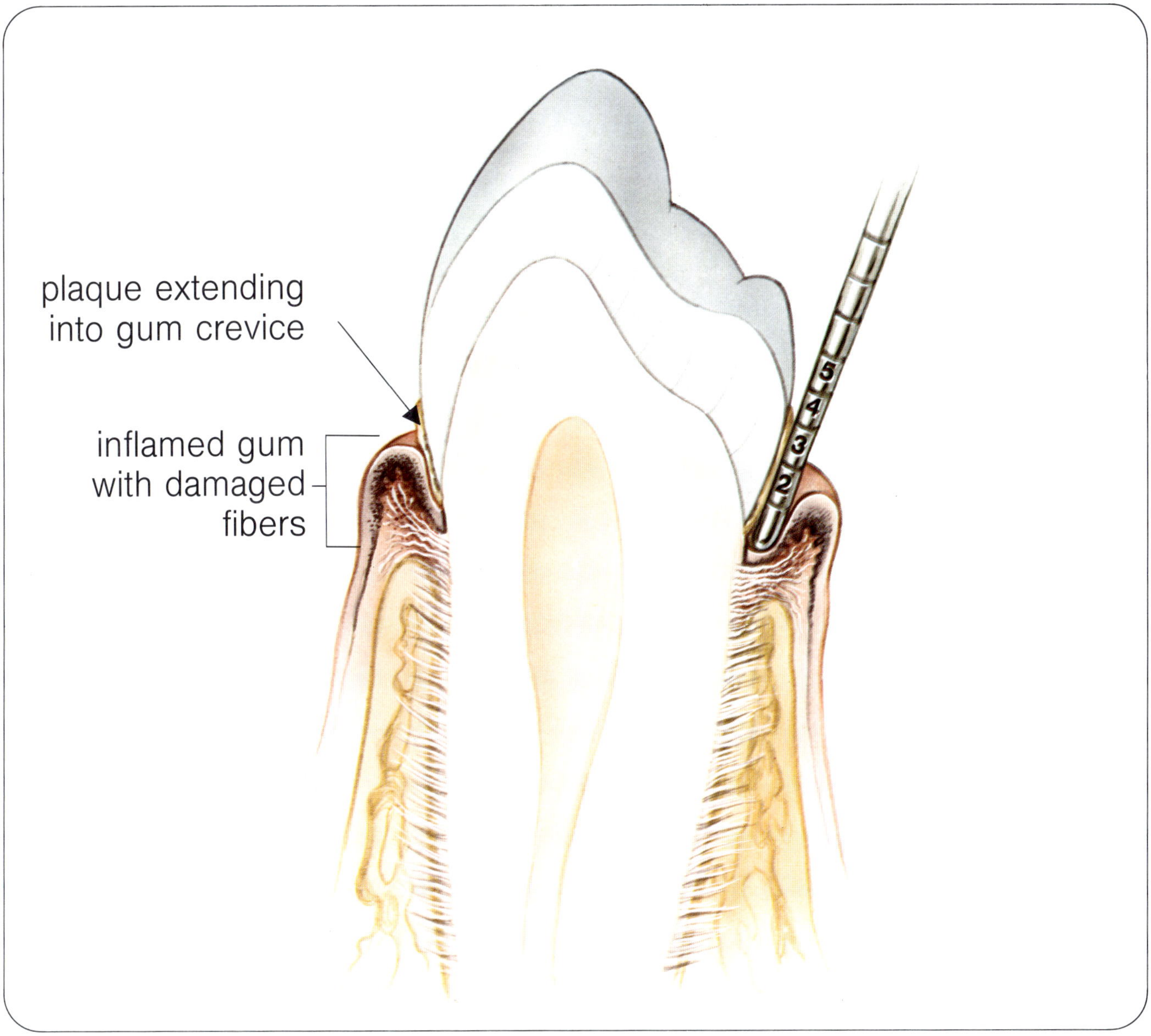

STAGE ONE OF THE DISEASE

Plaque has caused inflammation: the gum is red and swollen.

Inflammation damages the periodontal fibers that hold the gum tight against the tooth. This allows plaque to enter deeper into the gum crevice where it can do even more damage.

Proper treatment and good home care at this earliest stage usually stop the disease completely. The gums restore themselves to full health, with no permanent damage.

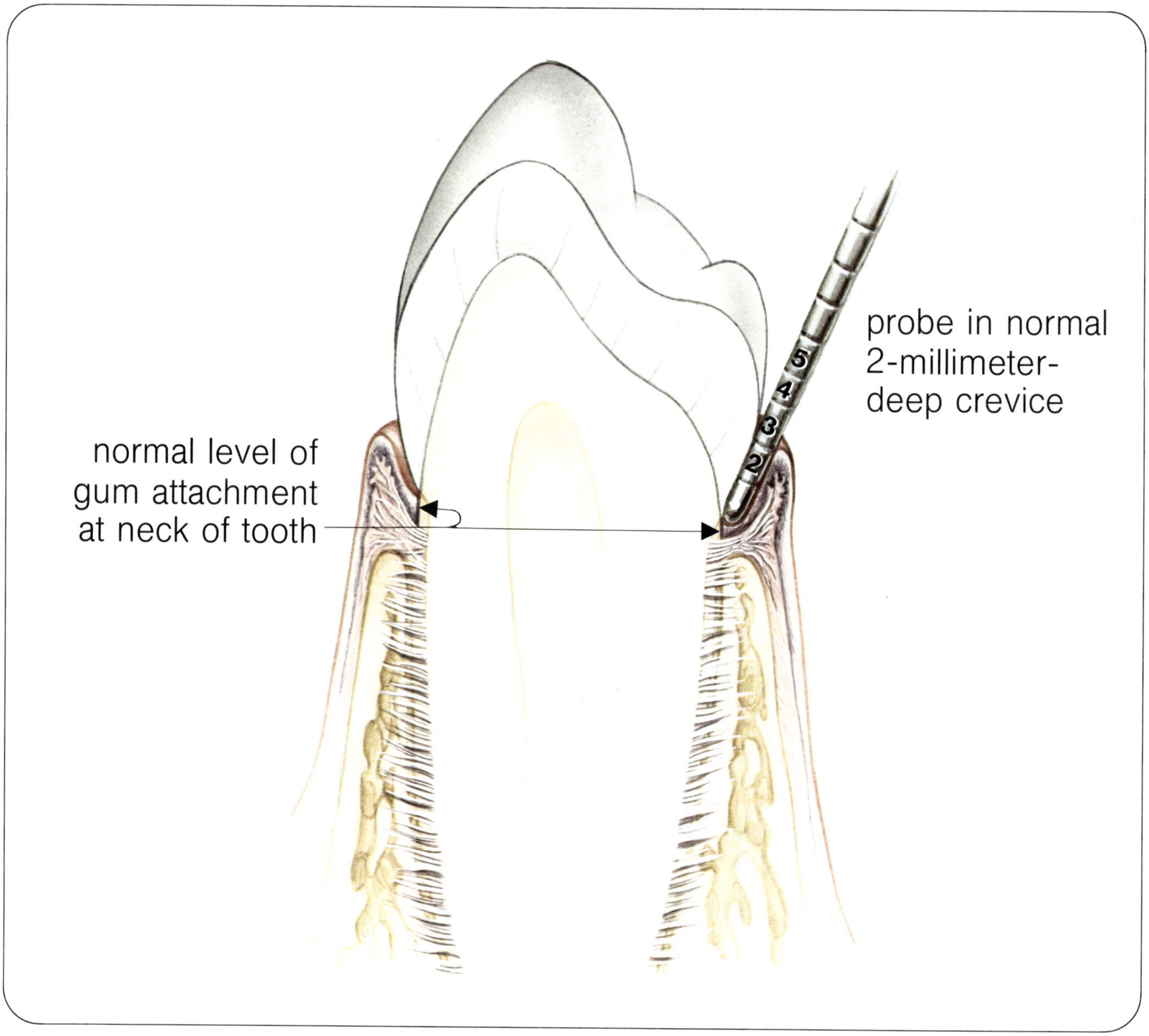

THE NORMAL

STAGE TWO (opposite page)

If plaque irritation persists, it causes the *attachment of the gum to move down the root*. This "creeping" of the gum attachment makes the crevice deeper.

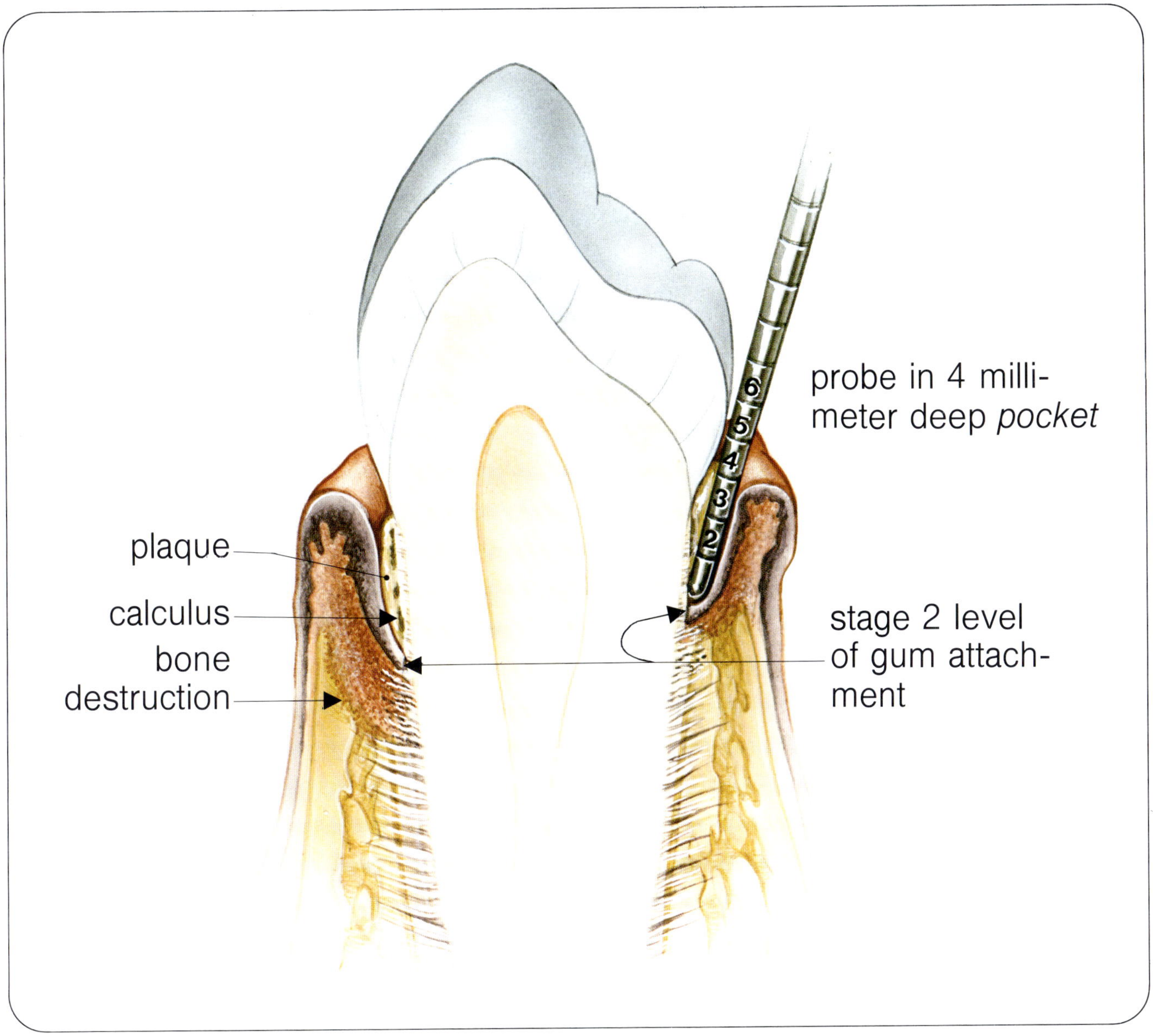

A crevice more than 3 mm. deep is considered a *gum pocket*.

Gum pockets are bad because they are very hard to keep clean. They are impossible to keep clean once some calculus has formed within them.

The toxins (poisons) from the plaque in this 4-millimeter-deep pocket have also destroyed some adjacent bone.

Treatment, plus good home care, will slow down or stop progress of the disease at this stage. But it is unlikely that the gum and bone can be completely restored to the way they were before the disease started.

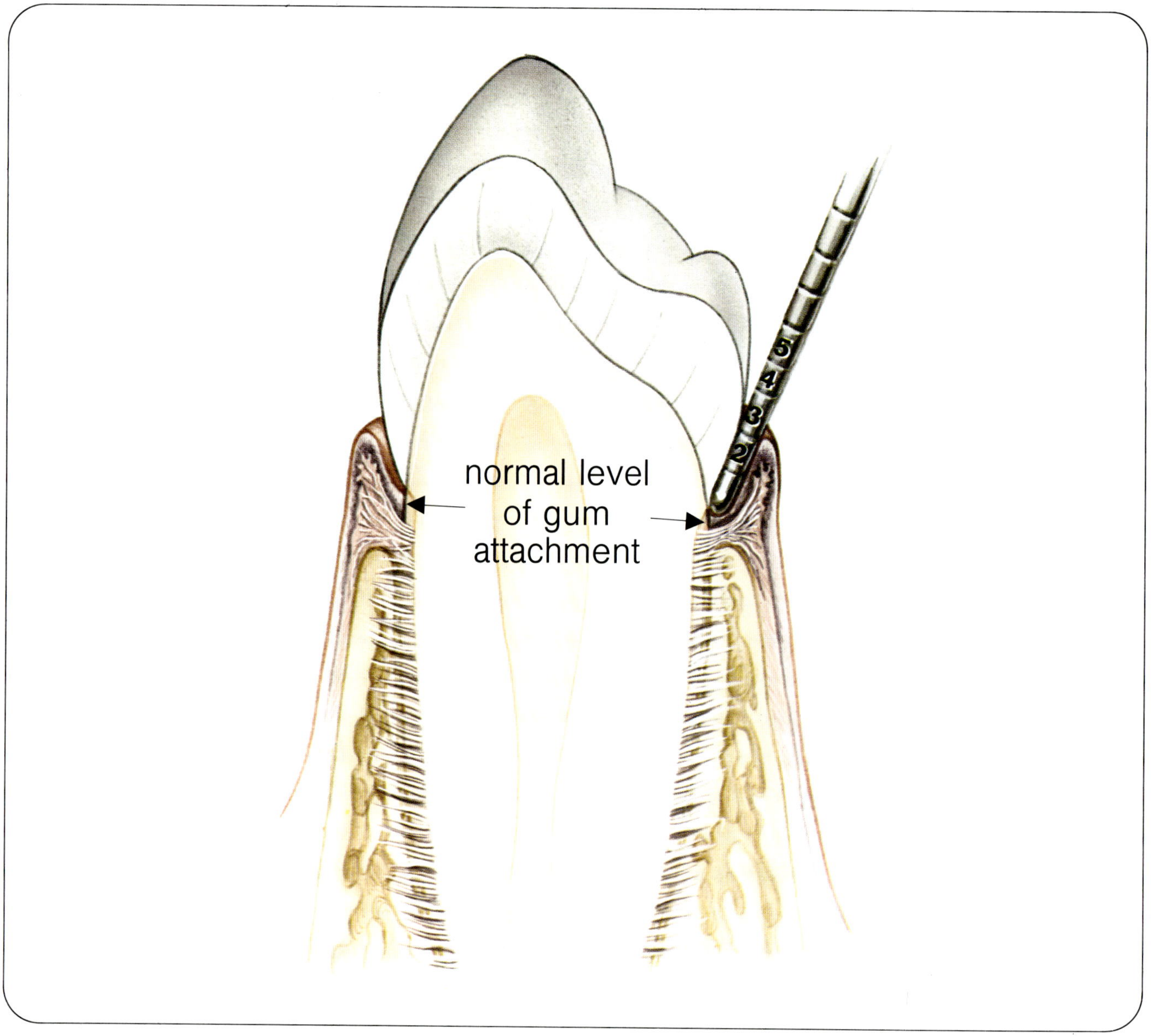

THE NORMAL

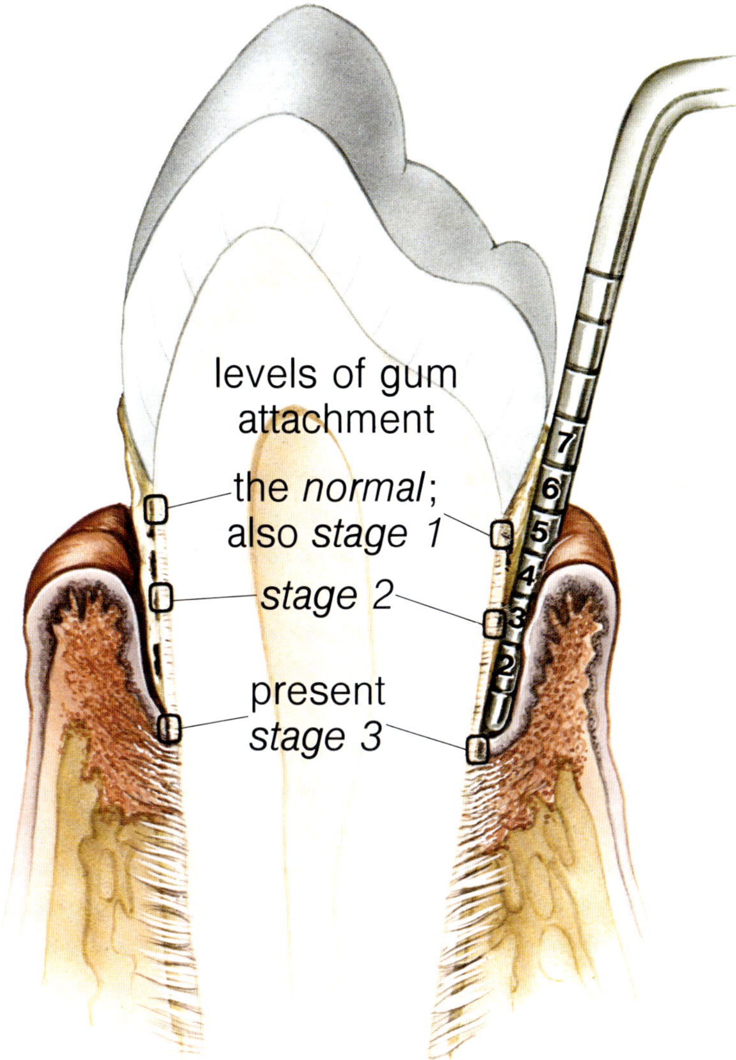

STAGE THREE

Continuing plaque irritation has caused the loss of more bone support, and the gum attachment has crept a little farther down the root. Again, treatment plus good home care can still stop the progress of disease at this stage.

Pus forms in pockets like these and escapes into the mouth to cause *bad breath*.

STAGE FOUR (opposite)

Half the original bone holding the tooth has been lost.

Chewing on teeth with so little bone support puts tremendous stress on bone that remains, and causes still faster bone loss.

Note how far the margin of the gum has withdrawn down the root. This *receding of the gums* exposes part of the root and makes the tooth look longer when seen in the mouth.

Even in this advanced stage of periodontal disease, treatment and proper home care usually help considerably.

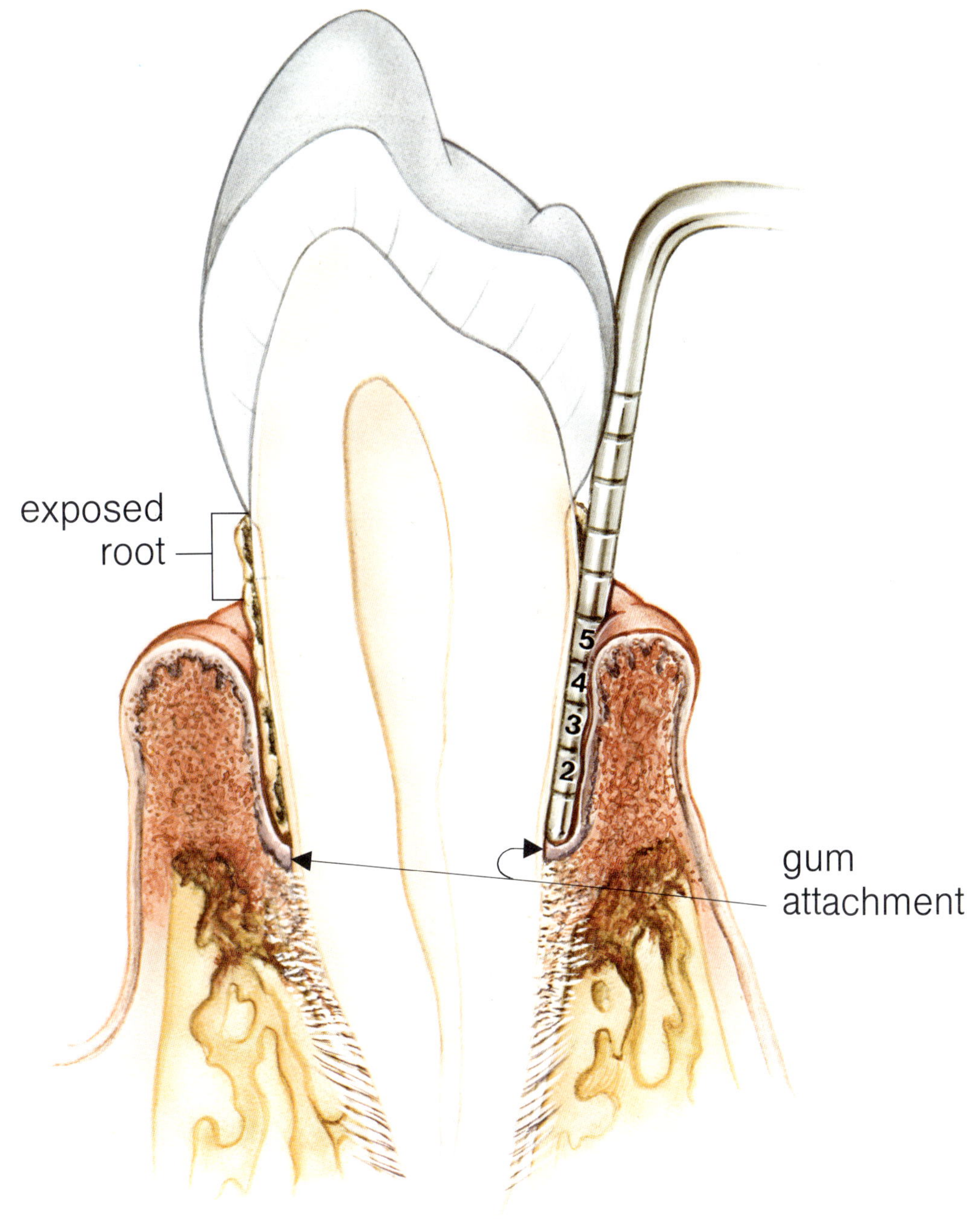
exposed
root
5
4
3
2
gum
attachment

The diagram on the opposite page dramatically shows how much bone loss and gum recession have taken place at STAGE FOUR.

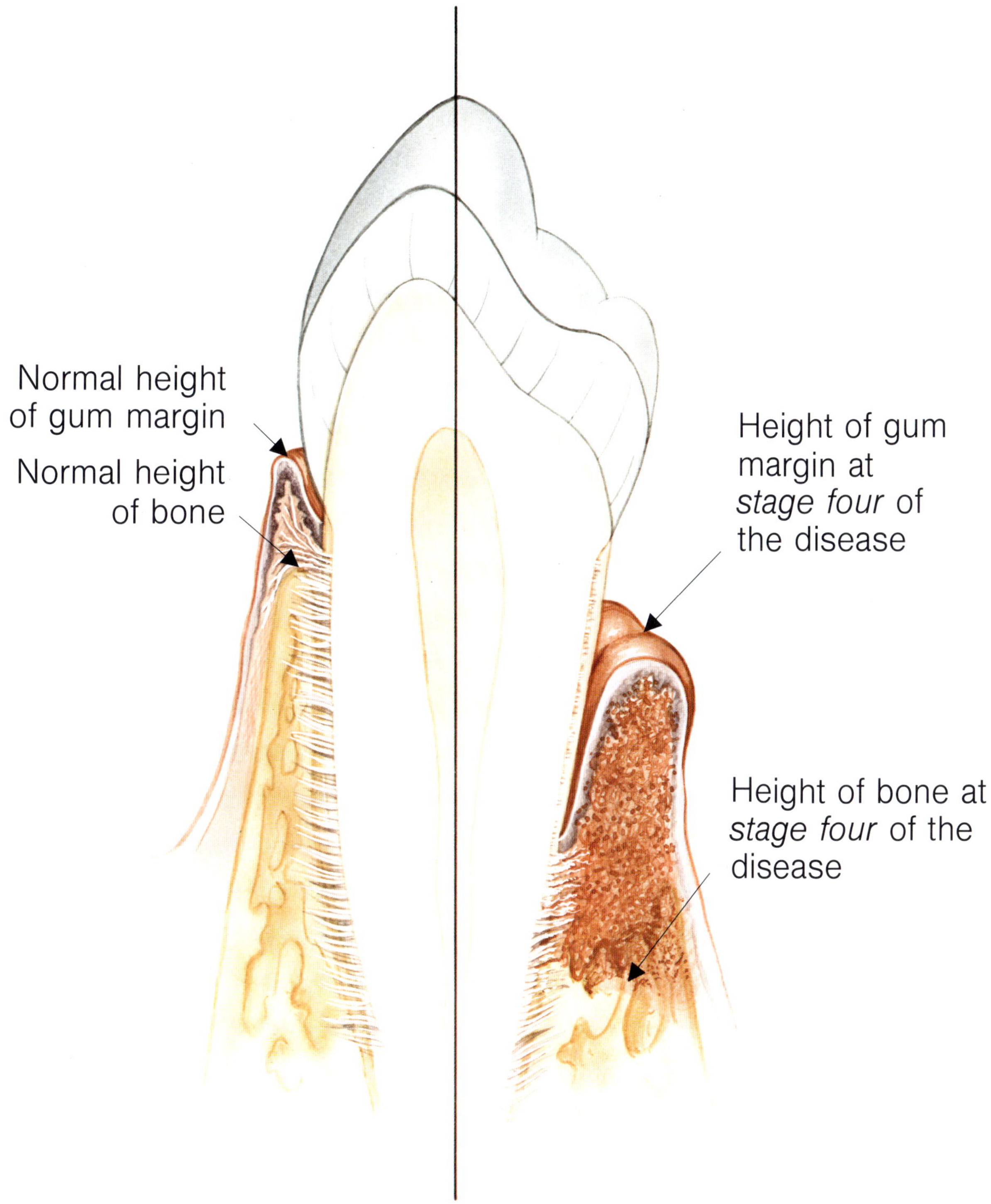
Normal height
of gum margin
Normal height
of bone
Height of gum
margin at
stage four of
the disease
Height of bone at
stage four of the
disease

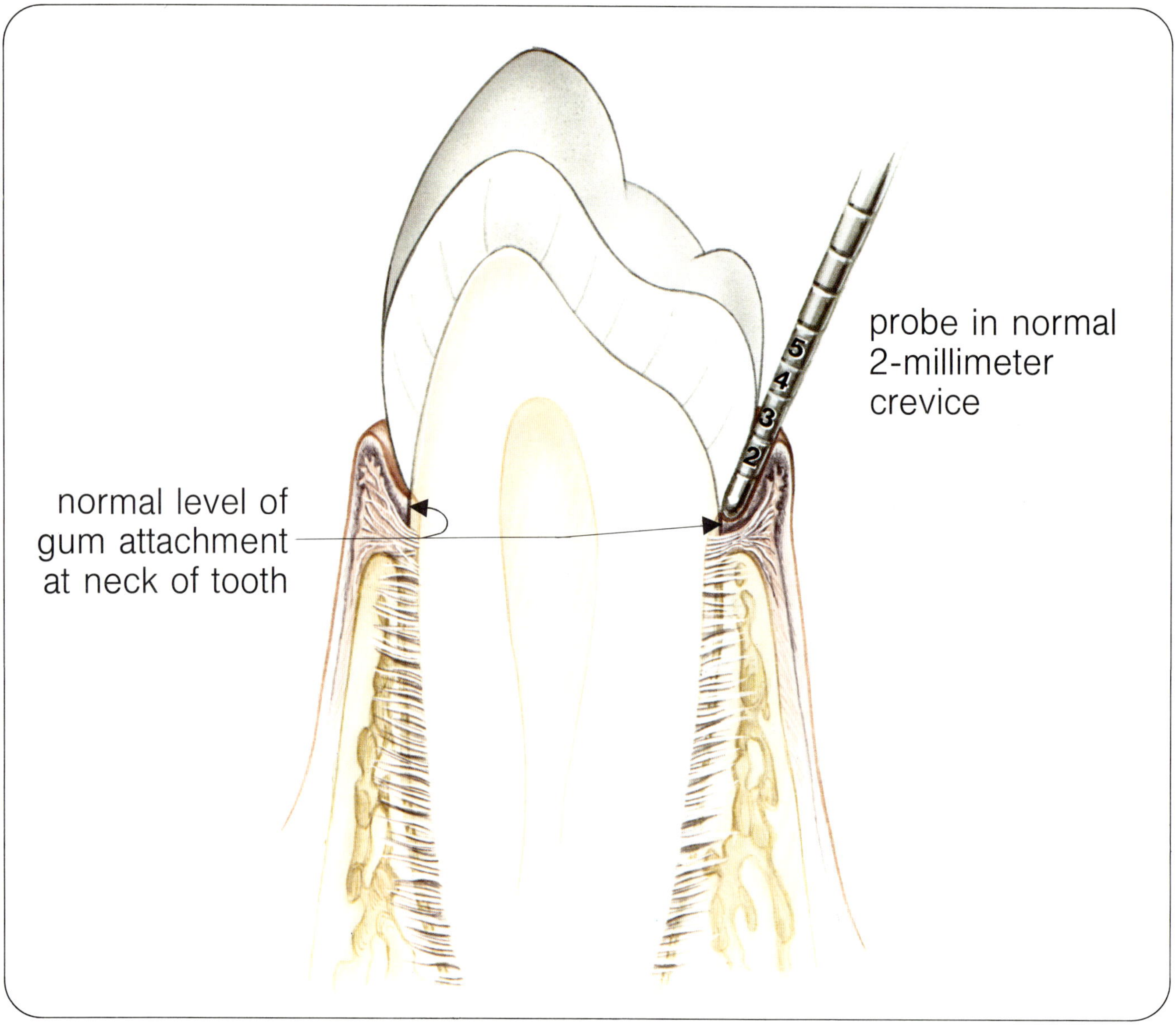
probe in normal
2-millimeter
crevice
5
4
3
2
normal level of
gum attachment
at neck of tooth

THE NORMAL

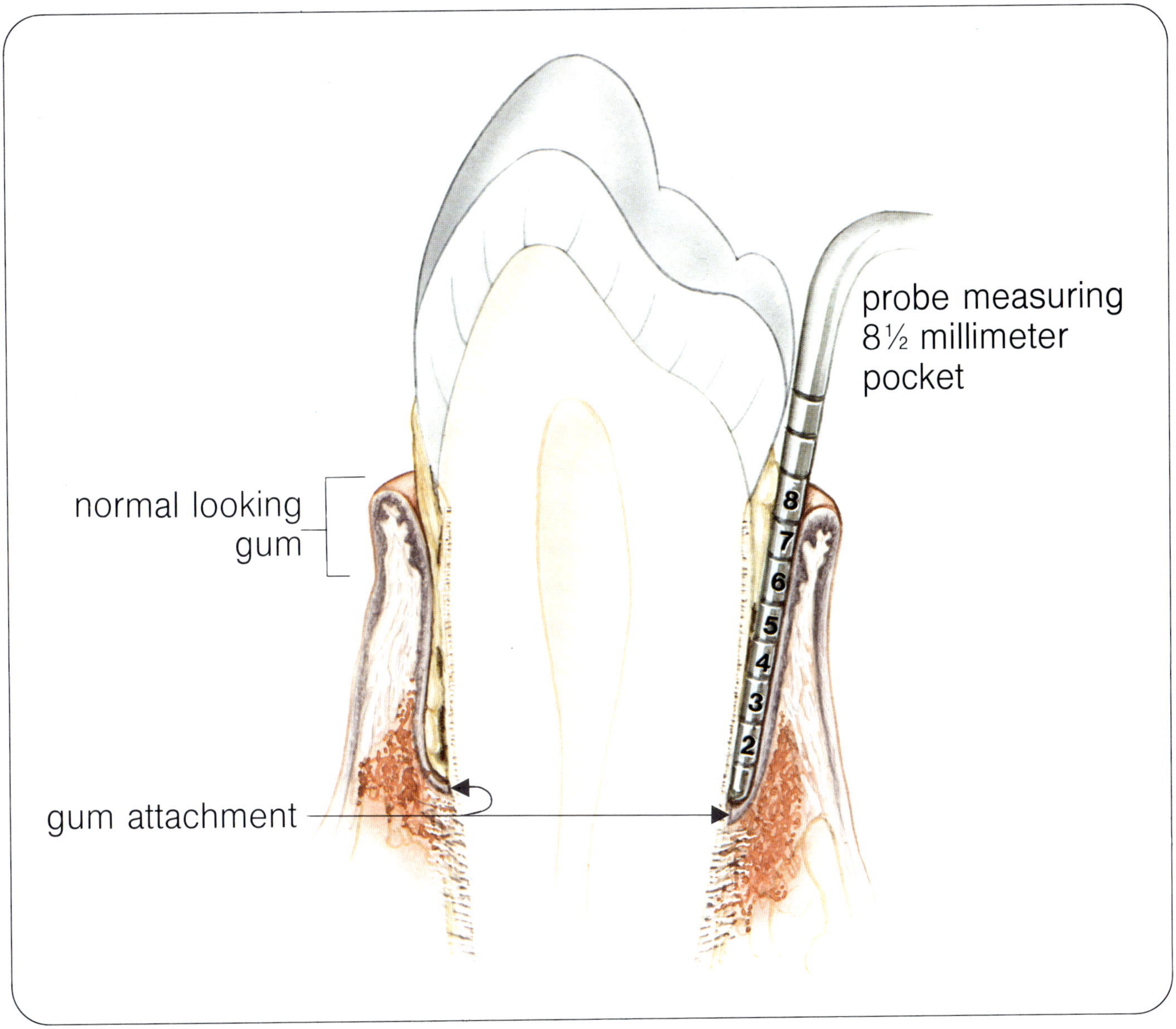

A DECEIVING VARIATION OF PERIODONTAL DISEASE

The *gum attachment* here is at the same level as in the STAGE FOUR diagram on page 63. But here the gum is so enlarged from long-standing disease it *still hides the root*. There is disease at the bottom of the pocket, far from the upper edges of the gum. These gums would look rather normal to the untrained observer.

This situation could fool you into thinking everything is all right.

A dentist would find this pocket during a routine periodontal examination.

STAGE FIVE (opposite)

Now it is too late for any treatment. Not enough bone remains, and the inflammation surrounds the entire root end. The tooth is very loose. If your dentist does not extract it, it will eventually fall out.

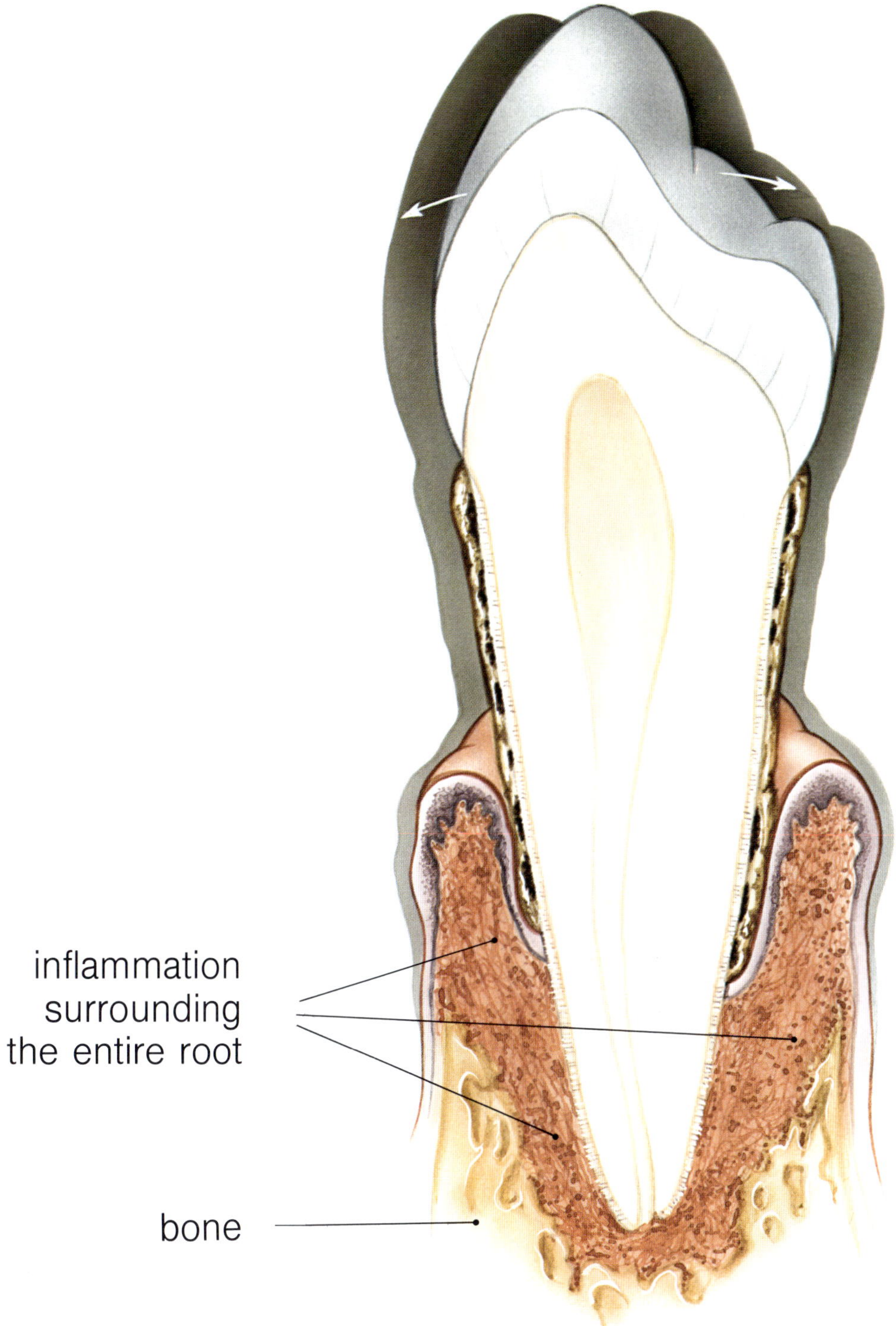
inflammation
surrounding
the entire root
bone

CONCLUSIONS OF PART II

Plaque bacteria produce the *toxins* that cause periodontal disease.

If untreated, periodontal disease can cause *bone loss* and *receding gums*.

If periodontal disease destroys enough of the bone supporting a tooth, you will lose the tooth.

Periodontal disease need not happen:

Brush and floss properly to remove all the plaque.
Get regular periodontal examinations.
Follow through on any necessary treatment.